1980

Sister M. ___

A New Approach to Medicine

A New Approach to Medicine

Principles and Priorities in Health Care

by

JOHN FRY

Family Practitioner and WHO Consultant

University Park Press
Baltimore

Published in USA and Canada by
University Park Press,
233 East Redwood Street
Baltimore, Maryland 21202

Published in UK by
MTP Press Limited
St Leonard's House
Lancaster, Lancs.

Library of Congress Cataloging in Publication Data

Fry, John, 1922
  A new approach to medicine.

  Includes index.
  1. Medical care.   I. Title.

RA393.F78   362.1
ISBN 0-8391-1282-3   LCC 78-6056

Printed in Great Britain

Contents

Preface

Medicine is news. There is constant public interest in health and disease; in medical miracles and in breakthroughs; in medical disasters, failures and malpraxis; in deficiencies and defects of health services; and in the rising costs of health care.

Medicine is 'big business'. Physicians come out near the top money earners in most medical care systems. In the United Kingdom the National Health Service (NHS) now costs over £6000 million a year ($10 800 million), a free service that costs every British man, woman and child £120 a year ($216) in direct and indirect taxes. But this is less than the £500 ($900) a year that medical care costs each person in USA and West Germany. In developed countries health care costs are approaching 10% of the gross national product (GNP). It is big business also in that in Britain the NHS is one of the largest employers; about 1 million Britons work as employees of the NHS, caring for the other 54 millions and in the USA the numbers are 5 million caring for 2.5 millions.

The provision of health services is full of problems and dilemmas. These problems and dilemmas cross all national boundaries. All countries share the same problems and dilemmas. Problems of objectives, of standards, of effectiveness and efficiency, and problems of relations between the medical profession, the public and government.

Medical care still is full of mystique. The medical profession still tends to be a great secret society, with many secrets. Many are secrets because so much still is unknown about health and disease. Therefore, many therapies and lines of treatment and management must be based on unsound premises. Much crazy care is given to patients. Much care seems less than useful and some is potentially dangerous.

This book is the product of many years of active study and

thought on the problems of organizing and providing health care. It began with the preparation for the James Mackenzie Lecture of the Royal College of General Practitioners in 1976 on 'Common Sense and Uncommon Sensibility' (*Journal of the Royal College of General Practitioners*, 1977, **27**, 9–17).

My objectives in this book are to examine some of the common problems and issues of health care and to consider some possible solutions. There are common issues that all who are involved in planning for and providing care are concerned. Faced with the restrictions in the amount of resources available we all have to decide on:

how much care is possible?
how may priorities and allocations be fairly distributed?
what care is useful and what is useless?
who should be trained to provide care and how?
how much clinical freedom should be given the health professions?
what public responsibilities should these professions accept in return?
what controls and directives by planners and administrations are reasonable and tolerable?

There are no easy answers to these questions but a world-wide public–professional debate on them is well overdue.

Beckenham, Kent, 1978.   John Fry.

1
Health Care and its Problems

The Utopian naivity with which we used to view medicine and its roles is past. No longer can we afford the comfortable, but unrealistic, luxuries of assuming that the roles of the physician are to heal and of the patient to be healed and that their relationship is sacrosanct and must not be interfered or tampered with.

Such idyllic situations never were real. Always there have been problems of providing and paying for care and anxieties over its quality and effectiveness. But it is only in the past generation or two that we have had the courage to begin to face facts and realities and appreciate the difficulties and dilemmas of endeavouring to provide good care for everyone.

At once we come across the insoluble equation of health care, namely, that our wants always will be greater than our needs, which always will be greater than our available resources. Expressed in another way, the challenge for us all, users as well as providers, must be to decide what is possible, what is necessary, what should be done, how it can be done and by whom?

The issues of health care now extend beyond the medical profession. It is inevitable that politically and socially health care has become a major department and involvement of all governments, because it is so expensive and so demanding a public right and since it must, forever more, be part of everyday politics. Therefore, there will be increasing interest and involvement in health care and its organization, administration, provision and quality of service by the people, by governments, by politicians, by public and private agencies, by trade unions and by the medical and para-medical professions, crafts and workers. No longer has the medical profession a controlling monopoly of decisions and actions on health care.

It may be difficult for present and future generations of physicians to come to terms with these new situations. Important among these are the less important and less powerful overall roles that physicians have and will have, in health care and the increasing amount of scrutiny and accountability to which professional medical care will be subjected.

The physician is now but one member of a health team, albeit an essential member. No longer can he, or should he, work alone. From the solo primary care physician working in isolated geographical areas to the super-specialists in complex technological medical units, all physicians must now work with nurses and other para-medical colleagues, with social workers, with medical secretaries, and with administrators, if they are to provide effective and efficient modern medical and health care.

Since there has to be financial involvement in health care by governments and/or by sickness and health insurance funding agencies there will be increasing concern by them that they obtain value for their monies that they pay to the medical profession. They will seek to apply modern marketing methods to health care and this must involve attempts to assess the quality and quantity of the health care for which they are paying.

CHANGING WORLDS

The last 50 years have been those with an emphasis on improving human health and comforts and these have been attributed to scientific advances and progress. The scientific explosion culminated most dramatically in developing and setting off nuclear explosions and setting men on the moon. Our scientific orientated societies have associated medical care and progress with such miraculous breakthroughs. The 'man in the moon' outlook in a public that is better educated and informed than ever before has created more and more demands and expectations for better health and more effective treatment of disease and less willingness to accept anything much less.

More and more monies have been put into medical research of all types. New technologies, therapies and drugs have been developed. Medical care has become more costly and more specialized than ever and is provided by a whole spectrum of physicians, from the most super-specialists and sub-specialists, through more general specialists and specialoids to generalists. A medical jungle has been created in which the unwary patient will inevitably take some wrong paths and get lost with possible dire consequences.

It is more necessary than ever before for each of us to have a personal physician who knows us, knows the true state of the art of medicine with the risks and limitations as well as its scope and potentials, and above all, who is familiar with the calibre and intricacies of the local medical care system and who can guide his patients safely through the medical jungle.

Although there is need to encourage and support cold science in the laboratory, it is even more essential that it is applied carefully as a healing art for the benefit of patients in the wards and consulting rooms.

Unfortunately the optimistic enthusiasm of the media men has tended to outrun true reality. Medicine and its scope, even in the last quarter of the scientific twentieth century, has been oversold. Life expectancy has scarcely increased very much for middle-aged men over the past decade, and the volume of work in treating disease facing the medical profession continues to grow. We are in danger of creating an over-expectant public whose demands and expectations for better health and care cannot be met. We must temper the science of the impossible with the art of the possible.

HEALTH

Personal health is the goal that we all endeavour to achieve and maintain and health care is the system through which it is carried out hopefully. In most societies health and health care are considered as human rights to be provided by others with as little personal effort and responsibility as possible by the individual.

But what is health? The definition of health by the World Health Organization (WHO), 'a state of complete physical, mental and social well-being and not merely an absence of disease', is a situation that is rarely achieved by any for any length of time. Health is a rare subjective state of mind and an even more rare objective physical state.

Applying the WHO definition to random samples of populations it seems that at any time less than 10% are 'healthy' and that 90%

3

are in a state of active 'non-health' though not suffering from overt diseases (Dunnell and Cartwright, 1972; Wadsworth, Butterfield and Blaney, 1971).

NON-HEALTH

In a typical year about nine out of ten will suffer one or more illness or accident. Of these at least three out of four will be self-treated. However, in a developed society such as in Europe or North America approximately two-thirds of the population will consult a physician annually. This physician may be a family physician or a hospital doctor.

Of the population in the UK (and the figures are similar in USA and other European countries), around 10–12% will be admitted to a hospital ward, 15–17% will be referred to specialist consultants in hospitals and clinics and 18–20% will take themselves, or be taken, to hospital accident-emergency departments. Taken as a whole it is likely that one-third of a developed society's population will receive hospital or specialist care in any year for non-health problems and diseases.

INDICES OF HEALTH AND DISEASE

The battery of statistical indices and data on health and non-health and vital statistics in developed countries show common trends. Birth rates are falling, people are living longer, the proportions of elderly people are increasing (to 10–20% of the populations) and the proportions of handicapped and disabled are increasing because of medical salvage. Infant mortality and maternal mortality have continued to decline and are good indicators of social and medical advancement. Yet there are no signs of decline in overall morbidity or in use of medical resources.

The quantity of life has grown and become extended but there is less certainty of the quality of health.

WHOSE RESPONSIBILITIES?

Our endeavours to achieve and maintain health, prevent disease and deal with it when it occurs demand a joint effort from providers and consumers. Responsibilities have to be shared. The individual, the family, the local community and the nation (state) all have their parts to play.

Promotion of good health and control and management of disease require more than reasonable medical resources, within which the health professions play their part. The individual has to be prepared to follow simple health rules and avoid self-abuse. He has to take regular exercise, a reasonable diet, maintain an optimum weight, and restrict tobacco smoking and alcohol consumption. The family as the basic social unit has responsibilities for providing self-care for minor illness and collaborative care with other health resources in more major and chronic diseases. Individuals and families have responsibilities in their selective, discriminating and economic use of resources.

The local community and the nation have the wider responsibilities in ensuring safe water and sewage and sanitation, adequate food supplies, housing, and in providing safe and satisfying work and rewards in a reasonable environment. They also have the responsibilities to promote preventive measures such as immunization and early diagnosis and treatment of disease. Such responsibilities are reasonable expectations in a modern developed society and if they were achieved then it is likely that health would improve and continue to improve.

DISEASES

Disease is never static. Within the affected person the condition may remain the same but often it tends to improve or deteriorate. Diseases themselves have certain characteristic patterns of natural history (see page 69). Some are disorders of ageing, that tend to become more frequent and more disabling as persons grow older. Some disorders affect children and then naturally disappear. Some that affect young or middle-aged adults have an onset, a peak and a remission. Some syndromes are most prevalent in the young and the old. Some, once present, remain unaltered until death.

Changes have occurred in diseases over the past century in developed societies. Diseases of dirt, deprivation and deficiency have become less prevalent. These include the major infective disorders such as tuberculosis, poliomyelitis, measles, whooping cough and streptoccal infection. These improvements probably have happened more from social than medical improvements (McKeown, 1976).

In developed societies certain diseases have increased in frequency, possibly because of environmental and personal factors associated with affluence. In this group are coronary artery diseases, certain cancers, road traffic accidents and chronic bronchitis.

Since we all have to die, if we live longer we shall die from diseases of ageing and these have become more frequent in societies where life expectancy has increased.

Another group of conditions is those associated with some inherited factors. In addition to the more obvious inherited genetic abnormalities there are disorders and disease tendencies and habits of behaviour that tend to run in families. The old-fashioned term 'diathesis' should not be despised or forgotten because it does depict a predisposition to emotional and psychosomatic disorders and disorders such as migraine, duodenal ulcer, asthma, and various skin disorders that are repeated in successive generations.

Then there is another group of common and well nigh inevitable disorders, 'normal abnormalities' in fact. We all have our share of minor respiratory infections, of acute gastro-intestinal upsets, of various aches and pains and traumata, mood changes, rashes and a number of other conditions.

A system of health care has to be able to provide care for all these diseases and for associated social problems as well.

CARE: PROBLEMS AND ISSUES

In striving to improve health and control disease through better and more medical and other forms of care we have tended to outstrip realism and have based too much on vain hopes, mirages, dreams and illusions.

Whilst scientific methods and efforts have been encouraged and supported in basic and clinical research and care, not enough hard scientific methodology has been applied to testing the value or benefits of all these efforts. As McKeown (1976) has noted a more critical approach to quality of care is necessary and we must pose questions: on standards (how well we do what we do?); on effectiveness (is what we do worth doing?); on efficiency (does what we do make better use of resources than available alternatives?).

With few brakes on restrictions on clinical freedom and with little thought given to costs and appropriateness of the therapeutic and investigative measures used, we have tended to adopt a 'gawdsaking' approach (For God's sake do something!), with 'crazy care' as a marked feature. Actions such as over-medication, particularly of elderly patients with chronic and progressive disorders of ageing, over-investigation using expensive and hazardous techniques, over-cutting, in excessive use of surgical procedures, and above all over-enthusiastic preterminal care that prolongs the final agonies before death, demonstrate the dangers of iatrogenic pseudoscience as a modern medical hazard.

Good personal care in our modern era requires more than ever before common sense and uncommon sensibility and it still requires the application of Ambrose Paré's plea made over two centuries ago, that we seek to cure sometimes, relieve often and comfort always, to which we may add that we may endeavour now to prevent hopefully.

Rather than go on with strident announcements of news about medical miracles and breakthroughs there is need to pause and con-solidate and even to engage in 'negative' health education, of both public and profession. We must honestly state that there are strict limitations to medical therapy, that many discomforts and disorders have to be accepted as non-curable although amenable to relief and that better health lies more in personal application of sound rules of health and environmental improvements than in more and more drugs, surgery, investigations and other forms of medical or para-medical intervention.

COMMON DILEMMAS

The problems of health care are international and intranational, across state, provincial and local boundaries. There is no single answer to every issue. There are some dilemmas that are shared by, and common to, all systems of care.

To repeat, we all face the insoluble equation of care with expectant wants being greater than assessed needs, which in turn are greater than the available needs. There is no system therefore where there is a sufficient supply of health care resources. The relative shortages and deficiencies emphasize the need for effective planning in making

7

the best use of available resources and ensuring wherever and when-ever possible fair and equable distribution, geographically and socially, as well as on medical grounds. There have to be priorities that should be spelled out and agreed and accepted by public and profession and some rationing has to be applied.

If a health care system is to work well and make good use of its resources then it is inevitable that some controls and directives must be applied to planning and to everyday work. Duplication has to be avoided and good standards of care that are also effective and efficient must be ensured.

Acceptance of controls and directives is anathema to an independent medical profession that cherishes complete clinical freedom in caring for patients but a compromise has to be arrived at because, as noted already, the high cost of health care which requires government or quasi-government involvement in meeting costs means that some controls and directives are inevitable and will not only persist but increase.

A *modus vivendi* between profession and administrators is necessary for any successful health care system. Mutual understanding is necessary from both sides and reliable and up-to-date operational data and facts are essential if planning is to be effective and under-standable. Such factual data has been missing in all systems so far and is one of the main reasons why problems exist in planning and administration. Data is required to show what care is being provided, for whom and by whom, for what conditions, how, where and when and with what results? How well are the services working? Is the care being given worth while and are the best methods and resources being used?

Research to answer such questions must be built into every system of care and collaboration in providing reasonable amounts of data has to be an agreed condition of service by the profession.

LIMITLESS WANTS AND DEMANDS

The wants and demands of consumers of health care resources are limitless, and are exploited by the public and the profession.

There is a vacuum of sophistication in health care. There is, and always will be, enough work for the medical profession. There never will be a state of total health for all where no diseases exist and where there is unemployment of nurses and physicians – assuming that there is enough money to pay them for their services. Once major disease problems are controlled – in the past these were the great infective diseases such as tuberculosis, poliomyelitis, diphtheria, scarlet fever, measles, smallpox, typhoid and cholera, and in the future possibly cancer – there will be no respite for the medical profession. Into the vacuum that is created will come flowing in a whole range of new and previously unappreciated disorders (Figure 1.1). Thus, since the major infective diseases have been controlled, into their place have come more psychiatric and psychosocial disorders, coronary artery diseases and requests for care of previously accepted and endured aches and pains. This always will be so.

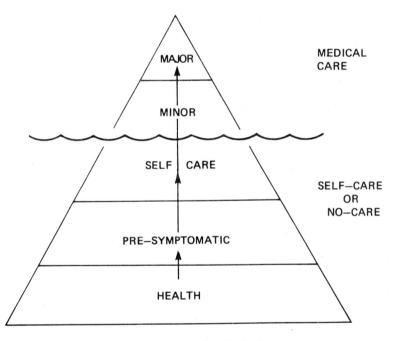

Figure 1.1   Vacuum of sophistication.

The British National Health Service (NHS) was planned originally on the false premise that once the major physical and social ills of the British post-war society of the 1940s and 1950s were corrected by new Welfare State, then the needs for care will become less and its costs will fall. How wrong were the naive optimists!

COST EXPLOSION

The experiences of the NHS have been that there is an almost bottomless pit of health care into which as much money and resources can be put and utilized.

The expenditure on the NHS has increased 13-fold in the 25 years, 1951–76, and even when reduced to take account of inflation the increase has been almost 4-fold (Figure 1.2).

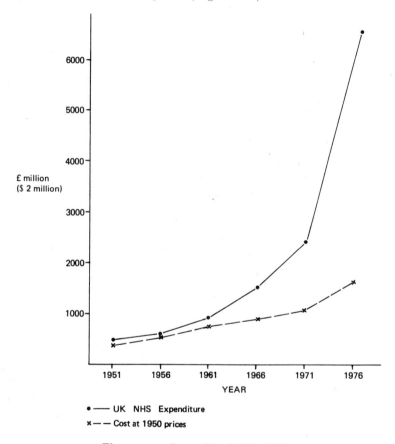

●——— UK NHS Expenditure
×—— Cost at 1950 prices

Figure 1.2 Costs of the British NHS.

Such escalation of costs of health care are common to all systems and they raise the question of how much any nation can afford to pay for health care. To what high levels can such costs be allowed to climb? How can they be controlled and by whom?

In 1978 the annual cost of the British NHS averaged out at £120 ($240) per person. However in West Germany and USA the annual cost of health care averaged almost £500 ($1000) per person.

HEALTH CARE SYSTEMS

There is no 'best-buy' single system of health care that can be introduced to and applied by all countries. Although health care is as old as mankind the concept of organization of health care is but 25 years old. Each country has evolved its patterns of health care based on its own history, culture, political philosophies, economics and wealth, education, religion, geography and resources. Evolution rather than revolution has been the keynote in which national systems of health care have emerged. Whilst it is difficult to agree on any grouping of systems, Bridgman (1972) has suggested a practical one based on administration and legislative patterns.

1 Countries of western continental Europe (excluding Scandinavia) and Latin America

The axis of administration is Roman Law. The hospital system is based on local government but there are also private hospitals owned by voluntary religious bodies or by profit-making investors. The medical profession is independent and combines private practice with fees from social security schemes. There are frequent disagreements between the medical profession and the social security schemes over rates of pay and conditions of service.

2 USA

Medical care in the USA is based on free-enterprise and individual freedom of action. A pluralistic non-system system has evolved. There is a mix of government involvement and it is estimated that 40% of health care costs are now paid by federal and state governments.

The hospital service is a mixture of private voluntary, Veterans Administration, community public hospitals and the federal hospitals. Personal care is on a private fee for service basis, many fees being subsidized through pre-paid insurance or through the Medicare and Medicaid schemes for the elderly and socially deprived.

The whole question of the future pattern of the US health care system is under debate and discussion, as it has been for the past generation.

3 Scandinavia and the United Kingdom (NHS)

These systems are planned at central government level, but there is decentralization to regional, area and district levels for many services in the NHS and to county levels in Scandinavia. Social security is universal and under it comprehensive hospital care and personal health services are provided.

In the NHS general practitioners are paid by capitation fees and by fees for certain items of service, and hospital physicians are paid by salaries on a sessional basis. In Scandinavia there is a mixture of payments through salaries and re-imbursed agreed fees for services.

Somewhat similar systems exist in Canada, New Zealand and Australia but there is less centralization of planning and the social security benefits are much less comprehensive.

4 Socialist countries

In the USSR, Eastern Europe, China, Cuba and other socialist countries the characteristic feature is the merging of all health care activities with a vast national hierarchical system in which primary care, hospital services and preventive care are combined (see Fry, 1969).

5 Developing countries with historic and cultural patterns still in force

There is a large number of countries with historic civilizations which are now classified as 'developing'. Their health care systems have to take account of their old roots in creating modern health services.

Thus in India, Pakistan, Thailand, the Arab States, Turkey, Philippines, and even Japan, the newer influences of Social Security and other schemes have to be adapted to ancient principles.

6 Developing countries whose patterns were imposed by colonial systems

Most of these are in Africa, south of the Sahara, but some are in Asia and Oceania.

The systems imposed were public hospitals that were mainly for the colonial armed services, nursing hospitals and health posts. Rural areas where most people lived were cared for by paramedical aides. The emphasis most recently has been to encourage self care and primary care in the rural areas rather than support more expensive hospitals and specialist services sited in the cities.

LEVELS OF CARE AND ADMINISTRATION

Whatever the systems of care, there are within every system certain common and inevitable service levels of care and administration with similar roles and functions (Figure 1.3). Using such levels it is possible to compare the ways in which the various systems organize such care and administration. Each level is related also to sizes of population and to the expected grades and types of diseases.

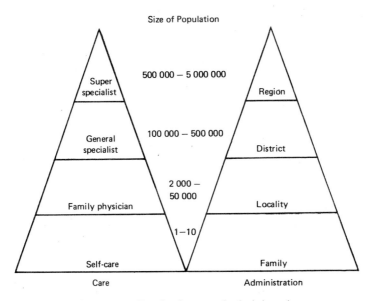

Figure 1.3 Levels of care and administration.

FLOW OF CARE

The flow of care in any system (Figure 1.4) starts within the family and then there are variations at each interface between the levels of care. Thus in the UK under the NHS there is in fact one single main portal of entry into the health care system, the general practitioner. It is he who controls the next interface when he refers his patients to specialists in the hospital service. In the USA with its more pluralistic system, the family has free access to the whole range of specialoids (paediatrician, internist, psychiatrist, OBG, etc.) and true specialists. In the USSR the family is cared for by the local policlinic, where the primary care is provided by specialoids, paediatricians and therapists (for adults) and in the larger policlinics there are available specialists such as surgeons, OBG, ophthalmologists and others. Hospital care is given by yet another set of specialists. In a developing country there is no choice and there may be no accessible services available locally.

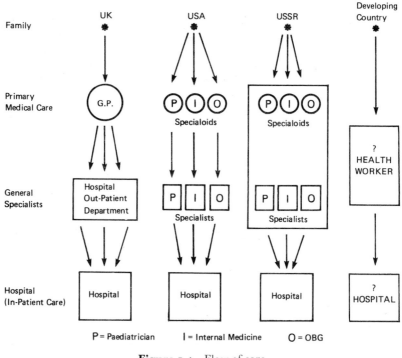

Figure 1.4 Flow of care.

BASES FOR A SOUND SYSTEM OF HEALTH CARE

Whilst certain minimal resources are necessary in any health care system there are other factors and features that require no resources and little expense that make for a sound system.

There has to be a plan with clear objectives and reasons for them. The plan has to be developed on reliable operational data and facts and their collection must have a high priority.

Once national, regional, area, district and locality plans have been produced it is necessary that extensive public education and information exercises be undertaken to explain the meanings and implications of the plans for everyone, the profession as well as the public. An understanding of each one's roles and responsibilities is important.

There has to be leadership, controls and directives, to ensure that resources can be employed usefully, economically and to good effect.

References

Bridgman, R. F. (1972). In J. Fry and W. A. J. Farndale (eds.), *International Medical Care* (Lancaster: MTP Press Limited)

Dunnell, K. and Cartwright, A. (1972). *Medicine Takers, Prescribers and Hoarders* (London: Routledge and Kegan Paul)

Fry, J. (1969). *Medicine in Three Societies* (Lancaster: MTP Press Limited)

McKeown, T. (1976). *The Role of Medicine* (London: Nuffield Provincial Hospitals Trust)

Wadsworth, M. E. J., Butterfield, W. J. H. and Blaney, R. (1971). *Health and Sickness: the Choice of Treatment* (London: Tavistock Publications)

Further reading

Bryant, J. (1969). *Health and the Developing World* (Ithaca and London: Cornell University Press)

Douglas-Wilson, I. and McLachlan, G. (eds.) (1973). *Health Service Perspectives* (London: The Lancet and The Nuffield Provincial Hospitals Trust)

2
Primary Care:
A Special Field

The level of primary professional care is a key to medical care as a whole. Not only is it a key but it controls the quality and the quantity of care at the other levels of care. Placed as it is between self-care by individuals and families and specialist care based on expensive modern technologies, it acts as a dominant influence on the use of resources.

Primary professional care has to exist in all systems of care and it has certain common roles, features and objectives. The systems may differ but within national and international variations these common factors are evident. Primary care has been a neglected field until recently. It has existed as long as health care itself. There always has been someone somewhere who acted as the professional of first contact to whom the sick turned to for care in the first instance. Yet somehow it has never caught the imagination of the public, profession, planners or politicians. It has dealt with the more common disorders that commonly occur and less often with the rare situations that rarely happen. Medical students, taught as they are in medical schools sited in large teaching hospitals staffed by specialists and super-specialists, get a perverted and distorted view of the community's health needs and this is in spite of the fact that about one-half of all medical students in all medical schools in all countries will become primary physicians, that is, providing first contact and continuing care to their patients.

There is no single prototype primary care physician that exists but in all systems he is recognizable from his roles. Thus, whilst in the UK the general practitioner is a clearly defined physician within the organization of the British National Health Service, in the USA the roles of primary care are carried out by a mix of family physician generalists and specialoids such as internists, paediatricians, psychiatrists, obstetricians, gynaecologists and even some surgeons. In the USSR primary care is very definitely organized and based on specialoid paediatricians and therapists (internists for adults) in urban policlinics and on para-medical feldshers in rural areas (one-half of USSR is still classified as rural). In Western Europe there is the tradition of single-handed family physicians working alone, although the trend towards group practice and partnerships is spreading from the UK to the Netherlands, West Germany and Scandinavia. In South America there is a great difference between free access ('free' if one has money to pay) to a range of specialists and specialoids who are prepared to give primary care; for the poor there are only the beginnings of an organized primary care service. Likewise in other economically developing countries early emphasis on hospitals and prestige specialties has created a relative neglect of primary care that now is being slowly corrected by training para-medical workers to provide primary care. All these workers may provide primary professional care that include many of the roles and functions to be described.

After centuries of international neglect of primary care there is now a sudden explosion of interest from planners and politicians. Headed and led by the World Health Organization it has been realized that primary care has a vital, inevitable, important and key role to play in economic, efficient and effective health care.

Economic because it is much cheaper than care provided in hospitals by specialists. In the UK general practice, although its numbers represent about one-half of all physicians, accounts for less than 10% of the NHS budget. If it can be efficient then primary care can protect the hospital and specialist services from unnecessary work. If effective it can restrict its own work to that which is worth doing.

WHAT IS SPECIAL ABOUT PRIMARY CARE?

For those who have not given thought to the matter, there is a need to make a case for the special nature of primary care and for special attention to be given to it.

Not only are the roles and features of primary care distinct and different from those of hospital-based specialties but its methods and techniques of diagnosis, care and .management of disease and problems also have a different emphasis because of the nature of the conditions and problems encountered (see Chapter 3).

Until recently, primary care has had no place in the medical curriculum nor did it have any solid scientific foundations or core of knowledge based on research. Now suddenly, over a decade, departments of primary care, general practice, family medicine, or other title, have been created, established and funded in many medical schools in the UK, USA, Canada, Australia, New Zealand, Netherlands, Belgium, Scandinavia, Austria, West Germany and South Africa. Notably, there have been no departments of primary care created in USSR and other socialist and developing countries.

If primary care is to carry out its key roles, improve, develop and expand then there has to be a much greater input into and support of teaching and research. Teaching in undergraduate medical education must include a period of special vocational training for those who wish to enter primary care and there must be continuing education of established practitioners. Research has to include operational qualitative investigations, experiments and trials to decide on the best methods and techniques of care, as well as clinical and basic scientific works.

ROLES

Primary care has many roles within a health care system. Above all it has to provide a reasonable available and accessible service to people when they first require skilled care.

Those working in primary care have to be trained, supported and encouraged to provide care for problems, situations, conditions and diseases which do not require specialist facilities or experience.

There is much more to good health and medical care than diagnosis and treatment of a specific disease. More than medication and physical therapies there are required total care of the sick individual and his family within the community. There are many social security services, rehabilitative and voluntary services and other facilities available in the community that can be brought into action to assist those who need them.

It should be one of the roles of primary care to instigate and co-ordinate the many and various para-medical community services that may be available not only for the individual's and the family's good needs but also to ensure that they are not misused or wasted.

Sound local knowledge and long experience should enable those working in primary care to manipulate the local services available to suit the individual patient's special needs, special circumstances and special personality. Different individuals and families may require different services and different specialists with whom they may relate best. It is the primary physician who has to select the specialist whom he feels will provide the best care for his patient. It may be that a patient with a duodenal ulcer may be best treated by surgeon A rather than by surgeon B, not only because of the surgeon's skills and experience but because of his personality and attitudes. It may be that a patient with a severe depression will be best referred to psychiatrist X who is known to favour intensive drug therapy rather than to psychiatrist Y, who believes in slow and long-term psychotherapy. It may be that Mrs M. is a proud and independent old lady who lives alone and who will soon need home help and home nursing if she is to be able to continue her independent functional existence at home, but her personal physician will be aware from the years that he has known her, that the situation has to be manipulated slowly and tactfully before she accepts the services.

It is false economy for a health care system to emphasize the specialist and hospital services and neglect primary care. It makes much more sense to create and support a sound level of primary care in order to protect the more expensive specialist levels from unnecessary work on inappropriate conditions. It is cheaper to keep people out of hospitals and in the community than to allow them free, or relatively free, access to the former.

Primary care has the role of acting as the protector of the specialist hospital services from inappropriate patients and as protector of patients from specialists and hospitals who may, because of their inexperience and lack of knowledge of the individual and family, undertake unnecessary and wasteful diagnostic and therapeutic procedures.

FEATURES

There are certain definable features of primary care that apply in most systems. In a district of 250 000 persons in a well-populated city there will be a large district hospital or perhaps two district hospitals providing specialist consulting and in-patient facilities. Within the same district there will be, in a developed society, about 100 primary physicians working in the community outside the hospital. They may work as solo independent practitioners, they may work in groups and they may work from a health centre or policlinic. However they work or are organized, there are the following features of the work they do and care that they provide.

1 Small and static community

In developed societies it can be reckoned that there is one primary physician to between 2000 and 3000 persons. This applies to the UK, USA, Canada, USSR, Netherlands, Belgium, France, Denmark, Norway, Australia, New Zealand and South Africa. Whether this is the right proportion is not certain (see Chapter 5), since it depends on factors such as work-load, methods and techniques and time available, but the facts are that this is what proportions are now and have evolved in all these countries more or less spontaneously and haphazardly.

In most places where primary care is established the populations tend to be fairly stable and static with not too much changing of physicians and patients. In the UK about 10% of the population moves house each year. In the USA the rate is double at 20%. In certain districts and places there is more or less stability. Thus in settled rural districts few persons move at any time, whereas in many large city centres there is a constantly moving population due to social insecurity. The significance of these two features – a small and static population – is that the physician and his team in primary care is able to get to know most of his patients well, particularly as in any year some 70% of his patients will consult him one or more times each year, and he will see representatives of 90% of families. Of course, where primary care is provided by an *ad hoc* system of the local hospital emergency room then no such stability and continuity are possible. Nor is it possible yet to achieve such care in developing countries where in some regions there may be only one physician of any type, primary, secondary or tertiary, to 250 000 persons.

2 Available and accessible

If satisfactory primary care is to be provided then it has to be readily accessible and available. The people have to be able to get to the primary care unit and the physician or other primary health worker has to provide a 24-hour service. There have to be primary care units within pram-push distance of mothers with children or old persons or there has to be a transport system or service provided or available to take the sick there when necessary. Attention must be paid to accessibility in planning.

A 24-hour availability has to be provided also. This may have to be provided by a solo practitioner but more usually cover is shared by rotas between colleagues or through commercial deputizing services.

3 First-contact care

Extra medical and socio-medical skills are required to make the initial diagnosis when a patient first seeks help. Not only are early symptoms vague and unformed and signs fragmentary or absent, but the dimension of time has not helped yet in defining the natural pattern of the condition. The primary, or first-contact, health worker has to be prepared to make a tentative assessment and diagnosis of the patient's presenting problems. It is no sign of failure or in-adequacy, on the part of the physician, to temporize and ask the patient to return in a few days for re-assessment. Because of the nature of the conditions encountered in primary care (see also Chapters 3 and 4) many will be transient, minor and self-limiting and many will remain as 'symptoms' with no proven or confirmed (by investigations) diagnostic labels – cough, backache, headache, dizziness, dyspepsia, sore throat and others must be accepted as such and providing that on follow-up they clear and the patient recovers then no further actions need be taken.

The primary physician is in an important position in relation to early diagnosis and assessment. He has to decide: what is potentially serious and what is minor; what has to be dealt with urgently, immediately and specifically and what can wait; what can be manage and what has to be referred to a more specialized colleague; what does he have to follow-up himself or what can he share with a member of his own primary care team.

4 Long-term care

Within a stable and static population the primary physician often provides care for his patients for many years and he comes to know his patients well and they him. This is a very special feature and benefit of primary care. On a typical day probably no more than one or two of the 20, 30, 40 or 50 patients that he will see will be *new* patients. The other 90% plus will be old patients whom he has known for some time. In fact, primary care is a continuing 'follow-up clinic' for the 2000–3000 persons for whom the primary physician provides long-term care. He comes to know them well as individuals, members of families, workers and local citizens.

Not only does long-term care help in providing good personal care it also gives the physician very special opportunities to observe and study the natural history of the common diseases that he encounters.

5 Content of disease problems

The primary physician can only meet and manage those diseases and problems that can occur in a population of 2000–3000 persons. These are inevitable epidemiological and statistical facts. He will deal with the common diseases that occur commonly and only rarely with those that hardly ever happen. In Chapter 3 the expected numbers are discussed but inevitably, and perhaps fortunately, he will spend his professional life-time managing minor ailments and helping his patients live with their chronic disorders more than in coping dramatically with the occasional major life-threatening situations. He will be asked by his patients to help them with a variety of personal and family problems and with a range of social pathologies that are not within the pages of the standard textbooks of medicine and which scarcely impinge on the work of hospital specialist practice.

OBJECTIVES

The objectives of primary care, as care in all medical and health work must be, are to 'cure sometimes, to relieve often, to comfort always and to prevent hopefully'.

It is important to stress the *sometimes* in an attempt to 'cure'. Most diseases, disorders and problems of human beings are 'non-curable'. They are, or may be, self-limiting, benign and short lived and are best managed by relief and comfort. Many chronic disorders of ageing and degeneration are inevitable and whilst greatly bene-fited by personal support and care, and relief by medication and other measures, heroic attempts at cure may cause more problems than benefits. Even with major life-threatening diseases such as cancer and heart diseases we must beware against making the therapy more grievous and unpleasant than the disease.

In our enthusiasm to treat or manage our patients be it for cure or relief or prevention, or give any medical advice that may interfere with normal life, we should always ask ourselves, as physicians:

1 Is the condition *normal* or a normal abnormality of life and to be accepted as such?

2 Is the condition *curable*, that is, how far should one attempt to achieve what may be impossible?

3 Is the condition *tolerable* for the individual patient? Tolerance of pain, suffering, disability, and discomfort are very variable and care and therapy must be moulded to individual requirements.

4 Is the condition *preventable*? Whilst it is right that emphasis be made in preventing diseases let us not impose unproven restrictions to normal life or add unproven measures in false attempts to prevent diseases. Better and longer life is most likely by following normal and simple health rules, such as: regular exercise; no smoking; moderation in eating and drinking alcohol; weight control; regular sleeping habits and avoidance of stresses. These are so simple, yet so difficult to follow, and so well understood by most people that one wonders how much time, effort and money need be spent on other unproven preventive measures. The medical check-up, screening of populations, fad diets, vitamins and other pseudo-measures have little sound basis for use in health care.

Objectives can be related also to what primary care can achieve for the individual, the family, the community and the nation.

For the individual primary care should offer a continuing personal service by a primary health team that may include physician, nurse and social worker. Self-care, self-help and self-responsibility for health and disease prevention must be encouraged through a form of continuing personal health education of patients whenever they have contact with the primary care team. Patients will be helped, educated and trained to make proper and best use of health resources. Attempts must be made to deal with the whole person and his (or her) problems and this is easier in the context of primary care because of our knowledge of our patients.

The family must be cared for as the basic social unit and the broad pathologies of family life must be appreciated and understood. They relate to the interpersonal relations of all who comprise a family. Stresses and friction between husband and wife are potent causes of symptoms and problems in primary care and there is scope and opportunity for family physicians to assist in their resolution. Relations between parents and children may become strained and lead to stress symptoms in parents as well as in young children. At the other end of the age-scale the care of elderly parents, uncles and aunts or even grandparents is now a common cause of intra-family pathology with problems of what care and who is to provide for the elderly.

The objectives of primary care range beyond the individual and family into the local community. Within the community the primary care health teams must plan to work together and in collaboration and co-operation with other teams to provide a service to the people that is sound, accessible and available at all times. This requires arrangements for out-of-hours cover and close working together to meet emergencies such as epidemics and natural disasters.

Primary care has to extend the frontline of health care from the consulting room, the health centre, group practice and hospital into the community. Through health education bad personal, family and community habits should be corrected, environmental hazards put right and vulnerable at-risk groups defined and helped.

Within all societies and countries primary care services must fit into a pattern within a health care system. The forms and details of the systems may vary but within them all there are certain national responsibilities for everyone. Best use has to be made of national resources. Waste and extravagence must be avoided. To achieve best results there has to be a national system of data collection, analysis and application to discover what is effective and efficient and what is non-effective and non-efficient.

SCOPE AND OPPORTUNITIES

Primary care provides special opportunities to practice the art of medicine, to use its crafts and to add to its scientific knowledge.

In our scientific age it is more important than ever that the potent, and potentially dangerous, investigations, drugs and other therapies are used with the greatest care and discrimination. Never before has the medical profession had such tremendously powerful therapeutic and investigative armamenterium available to cure and relieve human disease and suffering, but with such growth in power and scope there have grown also possible risks and side effects. It is the duty of all physicians, but especially the personal primary physician, to be selective and careful in his use of modern medical machinery and drugs. Patients have to be protected as well as treated.

The craft of medicine has become more skilful. New and better tools for diagnosis and treatment are available and are being introduced daily. It is very necessary that the best and most appropriate modern tools and techniques be introduced into primary care and that its practitioners learn how to apply them. But we have to be certain that new tools and techniques are better and safer than the old before they are accepted into regular care.

Primary care offers a new-old field for scientific research and study. Old because it is as old as medicine itself, and new because of the lack of research studies that have been carried out. Nowhere else in medicine can the natural history of disease be observed and recorded over many years by patient documentation by practising physician naturalists. Nowhere else may the interpersonal and intrafamily factors be studied as they influence the onset and patterns of symptoms, problems and disease complexes. Nowhere else may the early effects of the influences of environmental hazards be appreciated providing that we are on the lookout for them. Nowhere else can the physician train and educate him better than by keeping his own personal simple clinical and operational records that he can review and analyse regularly the patterns of the diseases that he is managing and the people for whom he is caring.

Further reading

Fry, J. (ed.) (1977). *Trends in General Practice* (London: Royal College of General Practitioners)

Hicks, D. (1976). *Primary Health Care, A Review* (London: HMSO)

3
What is Primary Care?
Content and Implications

Examination of the content of primary care will provide some appreciation of what it does today and what it might be expected to do tomorrow.

In most countries the evolution of health care services has created similar patterns of care in hospitals and specialist practice and also at the level of primary care. The emphasis everywhere, until recently, has been on cure and care of established overt diseases and little planning and co-ordinated action have gone into prevention of disease and promotion of health. What has been done has been on an *ad hoc* basis with few trials and experiments to test hypotheses, methods, techniques and their results, effects and benefits.

If the roles and efforts of health care in general and primary care in particular are to be different in the future then careful examination of the present content of work and its method and technique has to be carried out critically and constructively.

FACTORS THAT AFFECT THE CONTENT OF PRIMARY CARE

It has to be realized that whilst the general nature and content of primary care are similar, each practice or unit providing primary care is different in some detail.

There will be differences influenced by local epidemiology and morbidity. Thus geography, economics and climatic conditions will create differing emphasis on the types and frequency of conditions and problems encountered. Tropical and developing rural areas will provide a different spectrum of morbidity and problems from those in a developed temperate urban area.

There will be differences in content influenced by customs, traditions and expectations of the public and the profession. Thus in some systems and places primary care physicians will be expected and encouraged to undertake care of patients in hospitals as well as in the community. In some systems their normal work will include surgical, obstetric and gynaecological procedures, whereas in other systems such procedures are not customary, expected or allowed.

The content of primary care is very much under the control of the pattern of the national health system and on the controls and directives imposed on the health professions. It depends on the resources and facilities available and above all on the methods of payment and remuneration. In a capitation or salaried system of remuneration the incentives and inducements for provision of extra services are very different from a fee-for-service system.

The content will depend also very much on what the physician sees as his roles and what he is prepared to undertake and develop, particularly in undeveloped areas such as preventive care and for special provisions for vulnerable at-risk groups.

PRIMARY CARE: SPECIAL FEATURES

To remind ourselves it is necessary to recall the levels of care and administration (Figure 1·3, page 13). The level of primary care and first contact care is sited in a locality or a micro-district. In a developed country there will be one primary physician to approximately 2500 persons. This feature is responsible for the content of primary care. It means that the content of disease will be those conditions and problems that can be expected to occur in a population base, or denominator, of 2500 persons. It is obvious then that there will be a predominance of the more common conditions and an infrequency of the more rare conditions.

Of practical importance will be decisions on which of the conditions of primary care are amenable to care, cure or prevention and which can be properly undertaken by those working in primary care.

ANNUAL VITAL STATISTICS

An insight into the dimension of primary care are the vital statistics that can be expected in a micro-district community of 2500 (Table 3.1). This shows the approximate numbers of marriages, divorces, births and deaths that may be expected to occur in a typical year in a typical western developed community. The primary care physician will become involved in the joys of the births and marriages and in the sorrows and griefs of the divorces and deaths.

Table 3.1   Annual vital statistics in a primary care population base of 2500 persons (from Fry, 1974)

Vital statistics	Number occurring per year per 2500
Marriages	17
Divorces	5
Births	30
Primipara	13
Infant mortality	1
Caesarean section	1
Forceps deliveries	5
Unmarried mother	3
Deaths	25
Cardio-vascular	10
Cancers	5
Strokes	4
Accident	1
Other	5
Children (Under 15)	550
Elderly (Over 65)	375
(Over 75)	100

This set of annual happenings is a composite one and applies to a developed western society. Similar numbers can be devised for a developing society where there will be more births, more deaths, and higher infant mortality.

SEVERITY OF DISEASE

Diseases can be graded as 'acute major' or potentially life threatening acute situations, as 'chronic' long-term conditions with some functional disability and 'minor' usually transient, self-limiting and with

29

no risk to life or permanent disability. In primary care it is found that at any time approximately 65% of conditions treated by a physician will be minor, 15% will be acute major and 20% chronic.

These proportions are those experienced in a typical family practice in Western Europe, North America, Australia, New Zealand or South Africa. In a developing society there will be a smaller proportion of chronic conditions and more acute major diseases affecting children.

CLINICAL AND SOCIAL CONTENT

There have been many studies carried out to measure and define the content of diagnoses in primary care. What they show is a very similar pattern in developed countries in Europe, North America and Australasia with some differences to be noted. Table 3.2 shows what a primary care physician who functions as a general practitioner in Britain and a family physician in Europe, North America, Australia and New Zealand, who care for a population of 2500 may expect to manage in a typical year.

Table 3.2 demonstrates some very important facts. It shows clearly and dramatically what are the common and uncommon conditions of primary care. Of particular importance are the small numbers of the specialist hospital diseases and the huge numbers of the non-hospital disorders.

Table 3.2 Annual prevalence of illness and other events in the experience of a primary physician caring for a population of 2500 in a developed society (from Fry, 1977; Hicks, 1976; Marsland, Wood and Mayo, 1976)

Condition	Persons per year
Minor illness	
General	
Upper respiratory infections	600
Skin disorders	325
Emotional disorders	300
Gastro-intestinal disorders	200
Specific	
Acute tonsillitis	100
Lacerations	100
Eczema-dermatitis	100

Table 3.2 – *continued*

Condition	Persons per year
Minor illness – *continued*	
Acute otitis media	75
Sprains and strains	75
Ear wax	50
Acute urinary infections	50
'Acute back' syndrome	50
Menstrual disorders	50
Vaginal discharge	30
Migraine	25
Warts	25
Hay fever	25
Hernia	20
Piles	20
Vertigo	20
Chronic illness	
Chronic rheumatism	100
Rheumatoid arthritis	10
Osteoarthritis of hips	5
High blood pressure	100
Chronic mental illness	460
Coronary artery disease (all types)	50
Obesity	40
Chronic bronchitis	35
Anaemia	35
Iron deficiency	25
Pernicious anaemia	5
Chronic heart failure	30
Cancers (old follow-up)	30
Asthma	30
Peptic ulcers	30
Varicose veins	30
Cerebro-vascular disease (all types)	20
Diabetes	20
Epilepsy	10
Thyroid disease	7
Parkinsonism	3
Multiple sclerosis	2
Chronic renal failure	less than 1
Acute major illness	
Acute bronchitis	100
Pneumonia	20
Severe depression	10
Suicide attempt	3
Suicide	1 every 4 years
Acute myocardial infarction	10

Table 3.2 – *continued*

Condition	Persons per year
Acute major illness – *continued*	
Acute appendicitis	5
Acute strokes	5
All new cancers	5
Lung	2
Breast	1
Large bowel	2 every 3 years
Stomach	1 every 2 years
Prostate	1 every 2 years
Bladder	1 every 3 years
Cervix	1 every 4 years
Ovary	1 every 5 years
Oesophagus	1 every 7 years
Brain	1 every 10 years
Uterine body	1 every 12 years
Lymphadenoma	1 every 15 years
Thyroid	1 every 20 years
Non-illness event	
Medical check-up (in North America)	250
Immunization	100
Contraceptive advice	100
Cervical cytology	50
Antenatal and postnatal care	40
Social pathology	
'Poor' receiving welfare	200
Severe physical handicaps	70
deaf	25
blind	10
Severe mental handicaps	30
schizophrenia	5
alcoholism	10
Unemployed	40
One-parent families	30
Problem families	15
Juvenile deliquents	10
Adults in prison	5
Major congenital disorder	
Cardiac	1 new case every 5 years
Pyloric stenosis	1 new case every 7 years
Spina bifida	1 new case every 7 years
Mongolism	1 new case every 10 years
Cleft palate	1 new case every 20 years
Dislocated hip	1 new case every 20 years
Phenylketonuria	1 new case every 200 years

What this table does not and cannot show are the human and personal problems and issues that are associated with many of the clinical diagnoses. It is not enough to 'treat' a new cancer of the breast in a woman of 55. It may appear as a statistic in a table but in practice it needs much time and care to help the woman and her family over many months or even years.

Obesity, arthritis, Parkinsonism, heart failure and most of the diagnoses noted will require long personal care. This is possible when the primary physician is able to care for a relatively small and static population continuously over many years.

DIFFERENCES OF CONTENT BETWEEN NORTH AMERICA, EUROPE AND AUSTRALASIA

There are some differences of emphasis between these three areas. In Europe, and in the UK in particular (Fry, 1974), the most prevalent groups in primary care are the physical diagnoses of common respiratory infections and emotional problems.

In North America 'preventive non-illness' procedures are the most frequently recorded in primary care practice, followed by common respiratory infections, high blood pressure, diabetes, heart diseases and minor trauma.

Australia and New Zealand come between Europe and North American practices. There are more routine non-illness preventive procedures than in Europe but the physical diagnoses are more akin to Europe with respiratory infections more prominent.

The reasons for these differences are not due to differences of true disease incidence. It is unlikely that there are so many more cases of high blood pressure and diabetes in USA than in UK and that there are so many more persons with respiratory infections and emotional problems. The differences are there because of differing incentives and expectations for care of these conditions. In the USA primary physicians appear to spend much more time with their patients with high blood pressure and diabetes than in the UK. The end results do not appear to be any different.

DIFFERENCES BETWEEN DEVELOPING AND DEVELOPED COUNTRIES

There are very great differences of detail and severity in the expected contents in primary care in developed and developing countries.

Some of the common diseases of developing countries are the same as those of developed countries such as respiratory infections, trauma, gastro-intestinal infections and anxieties and depressions but any similarities soon become blurred because of the great underlying factors of ignorance, poverty, prejudice and fecundity. Ignorance and poverty lead to poor nutrition, contaminated water supplies and inadequate sanitation.

The picture of common diseases in primary care in Africa, Asia and South America are not the exotic tropical disorders but rather diseases that were common in developed western countries in the last century. They are diseases of under-nutrition, communicable infections and vector borne illnesses, whereas in developed countries now the emphasis is more on disorders of over-nutrition, stress and degeneration. Common to both societies are ill effects of trauma, alcohol, drugs, venereal diseases and social pathologies.

More specifically primary care workers in developing countries are faced with more severe presentations and complications of upper and lower respiratory infections. Mastoiditis and rheumatic fever are still frequent. With fecundity comes a much younger population with a much higher infant mortality. Malnutrition, starvation and gastro-enteritis are frequent. Common children's infections such as measles, whooping cough, poliomyelitis and streptococcal infections are much more serious with appreciable mortality and complications.

In spite of these differences the most common frequent groups of diseases in developing countries are, in order: respiratory infections; gastro-intestinal infections; skin disorders; trauma; nervous disorders.

The problems of primary health care in developing countries are not those of lack of knowledge requiring more research but those of non-application and implementation of what we know already because of lack of money, resources, leadership and motivation.

IMPLICATIONS

The applications and implications of this content of clinical and social morbidity and pathology will be developed in subsequent chapters in some detail. Here, it is sufficient to make a few general points.

There will be important questions on what the primary physician can and should undertake. For example, surely he should not undertake surgery for the five, and only five, cases of acute appendicitis that he will have to treat in his practice each year. A potentially difficult surgical abdominal operation should, ideally, be carried out by a surgical specialist. However the primary physician should be more than able to manage his patients with asthma, high blood pressure, diabetes, epilepsy, peptic ulcers, arthritis and many others.

To do his work well the primary physician must have resources for investigation and treatment and these include access to specialists in times of need. However it is the primary care physician who should remain in ultimate charge and control of the patient's long-term care.

There is scope to provide better care for the vulnerable and at-risk groups of the elderly and the chronic sick. The elderly account for over 15% of the population in many developed societies. Some of the social problems were noted in Table 3.2. The cold numbers quoted hide much personal and family misery and suffering requiring care and support.

To provide good and better care an early requirement is a system of simple but reliable records to provide facts and data not only on the content of primary care practice but also details of people and their needs and facts about the methods and techniques used to care for them.

References

Fry, J. (1974). *Common Diseases* (Lancaster: MTP Press Limited)

Fry, J. (ed.) (1977). *Trends in General Practice* (London: Royal College of General Practitioners)

Hicks, D. (1976). *Primary Medical Care: A Review* (London: HMSO)

Marsland, D. W., Wood, M. and Mayo, F. (1976). *J. Fam. Pract.*, **3**, 23

4
Who Comes and Why?
Self-care and Primary Care

So far there has been discussion on what constitutes primary care and on the place it occupies in health care in general. Now it is necessary to examine some of the factors that influence persons to seek primary care and this inevitably requires attention to the process of self-care.

If we recall Figures 1.3 and 1.4 the interface between self-care and primary care is clear. The events and motivations that take place at this first interface (the others are between primary care and general specialist care and between general specialist and super-specialist care) are important in deciding on the extent and patterns of utiliz-ation of health care services and resources. Thus it is important that we should know about why persons seek primary care and also about the reasons for the variations that exist.

It is just as important to know about why primary physicians refer patients to other specialists and about the reasons that exist for the large differences between their referral habits (this is covered in Chapter 9).

The interface between self-care and primary care is a fruitful field for medical and sociological research. The subject includes topics such as the 'sick role', the 'process of becoming ill' and analyses of the reasons why patients consult their doctors.

The ways in which people care for themselves and their physician-consulting patterns are influenced by personal, familial and socio-cultural habits and factors. These habits, however, are amenable to changes in volume and direction. For example, the consulting rates of general practitioners in the NHS have been reduced appreciably over the past 20 years and in particular the volume of home visits has fallen (Fry, 1977).

Within my own practice the volume of work, as expressed by face-to-face consultations with patients, has halved since the 1950s (see Chapter 5). This has been due to a number of reasons but one of the chief ones was an effort on the part of the practice team to reduce the volume of work. It is quite possible to alter patterns of work in primary care and to reduce (or increase) the amount of work being done and resources being used, without endangering the health of the people.

SELF-CARE

Self-care is the true first level of health care and comprises numerically the major portion of the system. There are more people caring for their own complaints than there are attending health professionals. Self-care taking place within the family context dictates to a degree the whole pattern of health care. The better and more effective that self-care becomes the less, in theory, will be the need to utilize medical resources.

It is likely that less than one complaint in four is taken to primary care services (Horder and Horder, 1954; White *et al.*, 1961; Thacker

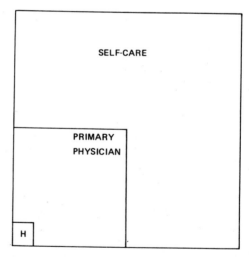

[H: Hospital or Specialist]

Figure 4.1   Extent of self-care.

et al., 1977). Morrell and Wale (1970) in a study of a selected group of women (age 20–44) found that diary records showed that these women recorded 'symptoms' on one day in three, self-medicated on one-half of the symptom-days but that only one symptom in 37 was taken to a physician. Elliott-Binns (1973) found that some attempts at self-care had been attempted by 95% of patients who came to see him as their primary physician. Figure 4.1 shows the extent of self-care and primary care in a proper perspective and also the small proportion of persons attending hospital.

On any day it is likely that over one-half of all people are taking some medication. Kohn and White (1976) in an extensive international survey found that at any time 27% were using prescribed medicines and 33% non-prescribed medicines (self-medication). The highest rates of medication noted were in the USA and Canada where there was up to 75% of medication recorded in NW Vermont, USA, of which 40% were self-medicating. The lowest rates of medication in the survey were in Yugoslavia, but even there it was 28% (10% self-medication).

Dunnell and Cartwright (1972) in a population survey in the UK found that over a 2-week period non-prescribed medicines (self-medication) were consumed twice as often as prescribed medicines, even in the context of a British NHS.

What is self-treated and with what?

The most frequent groups of symptoms at the level of self-care are shown in Table 4.1.

Faced with unpleasant symptoms few (16%) of us are sufficiently stoical and take no action to relieve the discomfort. Most (63%) will seek primary care advice and only 1% will attend hospital (Figure 4.2).

What do people take? The most frequently taken non-prescribed medicines recorded by Wadsworth *et al.* (1971) and Dunnell and Cartwright (1972) in the UK were analgesics, cough medicines and skin preparations (Table 4.2).

It may well be asked 'what were the results of self-medication?' It is not possible to give an accurate answer. Anderson *et al.* (1977) believe that it is relatively safe, does no harm and there is no evidence that it delays seeking advice for major conditions.

39

This piecemeal collection of facts still gives no clear answers to the original question of why do persons decide to seek advice from primary professionals? Why and when do they decide to self-treat

Table 4.1 Percentages of common groups of symptoms self-treated (from Dunnell and Cartwright, 1972)

Symptoms	Per cent
Respiratory	
Coughs, colds, catarrh, flu, sore throats	25
Rheumatic	
Aches and pains in joints, backache, painful feet	20
Emotional and nervous	
Anxiety–depression, tiredness, headaches	20
Gastro-intestinal	
Indigestion, bowel disturbances	10
Skin disorders	
Rashes	5
Others	
Accidents, cardio-vascular, gynaecological, eye problems, etc.	20

and when is the decision taken to consult a physician or other health professional? Presumably it depends on the nature and interpretation of the symptoms and on the habits of the individual, family

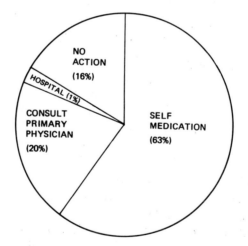

Figure 4.2 Actions for symptoms (information from Logan and Brooke, 1957; Jefferys *et al.*, 1960; Wadsworth *et al.*, 1971; Dunnell and Cartwright, 1972).

and community. They may consult because they are sick and need medical assistance. They may be anxious or they may need certification or some other help with social security benefits.

Table 4.2 Percentages of adults taking medicines in a 2-week period in the UK (from Dunnell and Cartwright, 1972)

Medicines	Per cent
Analgesics	40
Cough medicines	15
Skin preparations	15
Indigestion mixtures	12
Tonics and vitamins	11
Health salts	10
Liniments, etc.	10
Laxatives	9
Sleeping pills and tranquillizers	7

PRIMARY CARE: WHAT DO THEY COME FOR?

In Chapter 3 a detailed analysis of the content of primary care showed the conditions most likely to be encountered. This content of practice shows why persons come to consult the primary physician. In terms of broad diagnostic clinical groups the most likely ones are as shown in Table 4.3.

Table 4.3 Percentages of groups of conditions in primary care (from Fry, 1974)

Groups of conditions	Per cent
Common respiratory infections	25
Emotional, nervous or psychiatric disorders	15
Gastro-intestinal disorders	10
Skin disorders	10
Non-illness	10
Others	30

WHO COMES?

It is probable that the problems of consultations and health services have been studied in more detail in the UK under its NHS, where the populations at risk for all general practitioners are known, than elsewhere. Hicks (1976) in a wide-ranging collection of data on primary health care has some answers to this question.

Age

It is the young and the old who use primary care services most (Figure 4.3).

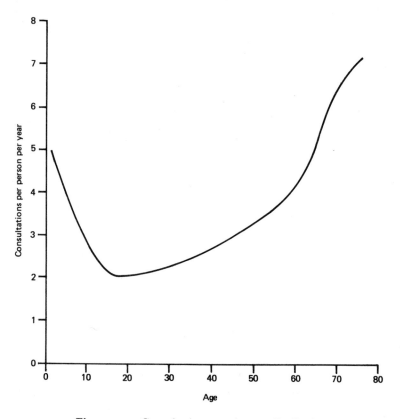

Figure 4.3 Consultation rates by age distribution.

Sex

Overall females have higher consulting rates than males, but baby boys consult more than girls (Figure 4.4).

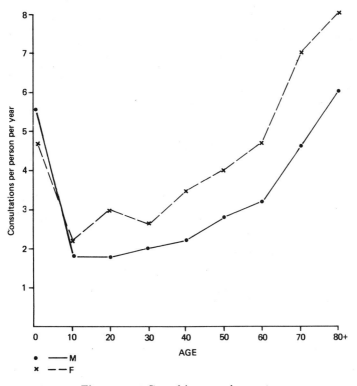

Figure 4.4 Consulting rates by sexes.

Person consulting rates

From a large number of surveys quoted by Hicks (1976) there
is a pattern in the proportion of annual person consulting rates

**Table 4.4 Frequency of annual
consultations (from Hicks, 1976)**

Annual consulting rates	Per cent
No consultations	34
1 consultation	16
2 consultations	13
3 consultations	9
4 consultations	6
5–9 consultations	14
10–19 consultations	6
20 and over	2

(Table 4.4). One-third of the population at risk will not consult at all in a year, another half will consult less than three times and less and less than one in ten will consult more then ten times.

Regional

In the two national morbidity surveys quoted by Hicks (1976) there were differences in the consulting rates recorded by general practitioners in the regions of England and Wales from a low of three consultations per person per year in the South-east and West Midlands to a high of over four in Wales. However, there was no regular pattern because neighbouring practices in the same region had consulting rates that differed by two-fold. It is quite likely that different rates of patient consultations represent patterns of physician-behaviour and control more than medical and social needs.

Social class and occupation

No great social class differences in consulting rates were noted in the UK surveys. The rates were lower in social classes I and II than in IV and V, with the highest rates in social class III (OPCS and RCGP, 1973).

The occupation that had by far the highest consulting rate was mining. Miners (and their wives and children) had consulting rates that were twice the overall mean and three times as high as the lowest consulting occupation, agricultural workers.

The reasons for the high rates in mining were not that miners suffered more injuries but rather because they required certification from their physicians for sickness absence, and the high rates were accounted for by minor illnesses which were used as a reason for medically certificated leave by the miners.

WHO DOES NOT CONSULT? THE NON-ATTENDERS

Each year about one-third of populations in developed societies with health care systems do not consult their primary physicians. This proportion has been found in the British NHS by Kohn and White (1976) in their international study and by reports from North America and Australasia. In my own practice I have found further that 10% of my population at risk will not consult me over 5 years and that 1% will not consult me over 10 years.

Who are these non-attenders and how do they differ from the more regular attenders? Kessel and Shepherd (1964), Baker (1976) and Anderson *et al.* (1977) have studied some of the features of non-attenders and I have done the same in my practice. Non-attenders are more healthy than those who consult their physician, but this applies only to major illnesses. They do not suffer any less from minor ailments such as colds, coughs, accidents and gastro-intestinal upsets. They are more self-reliant and self-sufficient and apply more self-treatment and self-medication than attenders. They have fewer expectations of the potential of the medical profession and of modern medicine. They are more likely to be men than women.

FREQUENT ATTENDERS: THE 'FAMILIAR FACES'

Almost one-quarter of the population consult more than five times a year in the NHS (the mean rate is three). Who are these 'familiar faces'? A few have conditions that do require frequent attention such as those who are seriously ill from acute conditions, there are those who are terminally ill and those with chronic conditions requiring regular and frequent supervision.

I have found that in my own practice the majority of the 'familiar faces' do not come under any of these categories. Most of my 'familiar faces' are persons or families who are more vulnerable socially and/or medically than the rest of the population. They attend more frequently for minor ailments. They are much more prone to suffer from emotional and psychosomatic disorders. They seek more out-of-hours calls. They have more personal and family problems and crises. They are more likely to be on long-term medication with psychotropic drugs.

These persons although a minority, probably no more than 10–15% of the population, require proportionately, more care and support. Usually their personal problems are either non-soluble or will improve on their own given time. Attempts at radical cure by the physician may cause more harm than good. This does not mean that sympathetic listening and psychotherapeutic support are not required, rather that the limits of care and cure must be accepted.

45

FUTURE OPPORTUNITIES

The primary care physician and his team are in a key position to control the use of services. They can prevent over-use and misuse by control and education, but even more important they should accept the opportunities to extend their care, involvement and interests into the community. Many of the reasons for seeking medical care are associated with social and medical situations that may be preventable, providing that they are discovered and medical and social measures used to remedy them.

References

Anderson, J. A. D., Buck, C., Donaher, K. and Fry, J. (1977). *J. R. Coll. Gen. Pract.*, **27**, 155

Baker, C. D. (1976). *J. R. Coll. Gen. Pract.*, **26**, 404

Dunnell, K. and Cartwright, A. (1972). *Medicine Takers, Prescribers and Hoarders* (London: Routledge and Kegan Paul)

Elliott-Binns, C. P. (1973). *J. R. Coll. Gen. Pract.*, **23**, 255

Fry, J. (1974). *Common Diseases* (Lancaster: MTP Press Limited)

Fry, J. (ed.) (1977). *Trends in General Practice* (London: Royal College of General Practitioners)

Hicks, D. (1976). *Primary Medical Care: A Review* (London: HMSO)

Horder, J. P. and Horder, E. (1954). *Practitioner*, **173**, 177

Jefferys, M., Brotherston, J. H. F. and Cartwright, A. (1960). *Br. J. Prev. Soc. Med.*, **14**, 64

Kessel, W. I. N. and Shepherd, M. (1965). *Medical Care*, **3**, 6

Kohn, R. and White, K. L. (1976). *Health Care* (New York and London: Oxford University Press)

Logan, W. P. D. and Brooke, E. (1957). *Survey of Sickness, 1943–1952* (London: HMSO)

Morrell, D. C. and Wale, C. T. (1976). *J. R. Coll. Gen. Pract.*, **26**, 398

Office of Population Censuses and Surveys (OPCS) and Royal College of General Practitioners (RCGP) (1973). *Medical Statistics from General Practice: Second National Morbidity Survey, 1970–1971* (London: HMSO)

Thacker, S. B., Greene, S. B. and Scilljen, E. J. (1977). *Int. J. Epidemiol.*, **6**, 55

Wadsworth, M. E. J., Butterfield, W. J. H. and Blaney, R. (1971). *Health or Sickness: The Choice of Treatment* (London: Tavistock Publications)

White, K. L., Williams, T. F. and Greenberg, B. G. (1961). *N. Engl. J. Med.*, **265**, 885

Further reading

Kessel, W. I. N. (1963). *M.D. Thesis on Non-attenders* (Cambridge University)

Mechanic, D. (1962). *J. Chronic Dis.*, **15**, 189

Parsons, T. (1951). *The Social System* (Chicago: Free Press)

Robinson, D. (1971). *The Process of Becoming Ill* (London: Routledge and Kegan Paul)

Stimson, G. and Webb, B. (1975). *Going to see the Doctor* (London: Routledge and Kegan Paul)

5
Work: Quantity and Quality – Manpower Policies

WORK: WHAT IS IT?

The volume and quality of work in primary care must be related to the nature of primary care itself – discussed and described in the preceding chapters. Consideration of how much work is being done, should be done and needs to be done, and how it might be done, are all important issues if sound plans and forecasts are to be made for our future organization of primary care, and health care in general. Primary care is a special and essential level of health care. Its chief features are easy and direct access and availability for first contact and long-term continuing care for a relatively small and static population base of 2000–3000 persons in a developed society. The situation is very different in developing countries.

The implications of these features are that the content of clinical morbidity, medico-social pathology and family and personal problems will be heavily weighted towards the more common and more minor conditions and situations, with a sizeable proportion of chronic conditions requiring long-term care and support. Most of the persons seen by primary physicians in such circumstances will be well known from a personal or family background and past experiences of care over many years. Very few will be new patients. In my own practice less than 10% of the patients who consult me are new.

NATURE OF WORK

The chief component of the work of any clinician caring for patients must be the direct personal and private face-to-face consultation.

This may take place in the physician's office, or clinic, or it may take place in the patient's home, or in a hospital or some other institution. The private consultation is essential to build up doctor–patient relationships and mutual understanding and respect. It is the situation where the patient must be allowed, and encouraged, to give a history of his illness or problem. It is the place where the physician can carry out an examination and make a diagnosis.

The most important component of any diagnostic assessment is the history as given by the patient, and further extracted by the physician. A physical examination, local or general, is a secondary process carried out by the physician but its limitations must be recognized. An examination of the patient is by no means usual or necessary for every consultation in primary care. Many of the minor conditions seen need, at most, a brief local examination. Many of the consultations in primary care (about two-thirds to three-quarters of all consultations in my own practice) are follow-up consultations for patients under continuing care.

Critical self-assessment is necessary of our own clinical habits if we are to avoid repetitive routine and stereotyped clinical habits that have been learned in the untypical situations of undergraduate teaching hospitals and which are scarcely applicable to the require-ments of and conditions in primary care. We must ask constantly the question of what for what? That is, what are we doing, for what reasons, to what purpose and to what outcome? New methods and techniques have to be learned and relearned.

The same reasoning applies to the next part of the consultation, the investigations. One of the characteristics of the clinically lazy and tired mind is to request a whole range of, or a battery, of routine investigations, often for no specific purpose but in the vain, and often forlorn hope that something may turn up from pathological and radiological screening processes. Although it has become a part of modern medical practice, the extensive use of investigations is not a criterion of good clinical care. By all means let us use the benefits of the modern laboratory and other investigative departments to help confirm clinical diagnosis and to assess progress, but clinicians must be masters of the machines and not their servants. In my own practice in less than one consultation in ten do I refer my patient for pathological or radiological investigations.

A diagnosis is the outcome of the consultation and this must be followed by a plan of management or treatment. The steps in the consultative process have to be followed in primary clinical care as elsewhere but with the conditions and situations encountered the process does not often require to be lengthy or elaborate. This does not mean that the methods of primary care are inferior to those of hospital specialist practice, rather that they have to be adapted to needs and requirements.

The indirect consultation is another form of work in primary care. It complements the direct face-to-face consultation. It may be a telephone consultation, more common and popular in North American than in European practice. It may be through correspondence or it may be the repeat prescription for the unseen patient (see also Chapter 8). The latter has become a major feature of British general practice.

Work in hospital may be a sizeable part of primary care, but the extent depends on local facilities and customs. It is very much part of primary care in North America, Australia and in many developing countries but it is not customary in Western Europe, Scandinavia or the socialist countries.

Administration, of necessity, occupies some time in primary care, but it need be a small part. A regular commitment has to be given to active participation in professional activities and continuing education.

WHAT FOR WHAT?

I have suggested that the basic contents of primary care are similar in all systems: so they are. What is different are the differing ways in which physicians tackle them.

Few comparative studies have been undertaken, but one is of particular interest. Marsh, Wallace and Whewell (1976) examined the process of consultation by 25 physicians in Iowa, USA, and by 28 physicians in North-east England. The conditions seen were similar but clear differences of management were noted. In Iowa the physicians undertook more examination, more use of procedures and instruments and requested more investigations. Many more were well-patient routine examinations carried out by the American physicians. The British general practitioners were more concerned with the whole patient and placed more emphasis on emotional and social aspects. There was more use of the practice team in care. The authors concluded that 'American doctors are more orientated towards a ritualistic clinical approach leaning heavily on investigation and hospital support. Their system must be expensive. English doctors seem to operate at a less definitive level of diagnosis.'

What the study did not measure was the outcome of care in the two systems. In spite of the differences in emphasis it is very likely that there are few, if any, differences in the recovery rates or other outcomes in measurements in the two patterns of primary care. More critical evaluative studies need to be carried out to assess 'what for what?'.

We need to determine whether ritualistic clinical procedures are useful and if so for what and in what circumstances? We need to know whether well-patient screening and batteries of investigations should be extended because they are useful in health promotion or because they are useful in increasing the physician's income.

INFLUENCING FACTORS

There are a number of factors that are involved collectively in work patterns.

1 *Volume of work that presents*   This depends on the population cared for, on the extent of morbidity and medical and social needs and on demands and expectations.

2 *Methods and techniques of care that are used*   Are they the most appropriate, effective and efficient?

3 *Time available*   How much time are the physicians and others providing care prepared to devote to their work?

4 *Resources available*   What manpower is available, medical and nursing, and what support are they given by hospital and social services?

5 *Outcome and quality of care*   These are the ultimates and the other factors must blend to achieve satisfactory outcomes.

DATA ON WORK PATTERNS IN PRIMARY CARE

There has been more data published on work patterns in primary care and of individual practitioners than of physicians in other medical fields. Reference will be made to publications from many countries and a constant pattern emerges. However, in comparing data collected in the various countries there are problems of definition and recording. There are also differences of detail in the work of primary physicians in different health systems that are influenced by administration, organization and remuneration. Providing that basic data are recorded, comparisons are possible. Thus it is possible to make comparisons on the basis of consultations (volume by day and week; place of consultation), hospital work, indirect consultations (phone calls; repeat prescriptions; others), out-of-hours work, administrative tasks, and time spent on duties.

PUBLISHED REPORTS

There follow summaries of some reports on work patterns in primary care. These serve to create a factual base.

Europe, North America and South America

Health Care (Kohn and White, 1976) is a publication of a World Health Organization team that collected data from three continents, Europe, North America and South America, from seven countries and from twelve areas. It is based on interviews with 48 000 persons. For a population base of 2500 persons there was a weekly volume of work with a primary physician of 210 contacts. The range was from a high of 300 in Buenos Aires to a low of 150 in Helsinki. One of the factors in this two-fold difference was the equivalent weekly contact-rate for other health personnel, such as nurses and social workers which was 200 in Helsinki and 105 in Buenos Aires, thus almost levelling up the totals of the two sets of contacts (i.e. 405 in Buenos Aires and 350 in Helsinki).

In the year of the survey 70% of the populations studied had consulted a physician. Of the doctor–patient-contacts 89% were face-to-face consultations. Further analysis of the contacts showed that: 65% were in the doctor's office; 5% were in the patient's home; 18% were in a hospital or other clinic; 10% were on the telephone; 2% were elsewhere.

USA

The American Medical Association publishes a *Profile of Medical Practice* (AMA, 1976). This includes data on the work patterns of various specialties and general practice in the USA from sample analyses. The American general practitioner in 1974 averaged 190 patient-contacts in a week in which he worked for 51 hours. Geographically there was a range from 273 patient-contacts per week in the East South Central region to 139 in the mid-Atlantic region. Of the weekly mean of 190 patient-contacts, 151 were in the physician's office, 34 were in hospital and only five were in the patient's home.

Riley (1969), in New York, reported a weekly doctor–patient-contact rate of 181, and Baker *et al.* (1967), in rural Missouri, found a weekly doctor–patient contact rate of 198.

USSR

In my book *Medicine in Three Societies* (Fry, 1969) I quote that in the USSR the primary physician is expected to carry out approximately 130 patient contacts (consultations) in a week of which one-quarter will be in the patient's home.

UK

In Britain, *Trends in General Practice* (Fry, 1977), the average weekly volume of face-to-face consultations is 175 (160 in the office and 15 in the patients' homes) plus another 50 or more indirect consultations.

Canada

In *The Family Doctor* Wolfe and Badgley (1972) report on the work of a primary care group in Saskatoon, Canada. The physician carried out 35 patient contacts each day or about 190 in a week. Of these 115 were in the office, 30 in hospital, 10 home visits and 35 on the telephone.

Australia

From Australia on *General Practice in Victoria* Scotton and Grounds (1969) report that the general practitioners averaged 186 doctor–patient contacts in a week of which 28 were home visits.

New Zealand

From New Zealand on *The Content of General Practice*, Lough (1967) reports a higher work pattern of 209 doctor–patient contacts per week of which 67 were home visits.

A PROFILE OF A WEEK'S WORK OF A PRIMARY PHYSICIAN

These reports also quoted the time spent by physicians in their work. Table 5.1 is a representation of the collected and collated data from these sources. There is a remarkable similarity in the volume of work as measured by doctor–patient contacts in primary care in developed countries. These contacts may be direct face-to-face consultations, at the office, patient's home or hospital, or they may be indirect (such as telephone) contacts.

Table 5.1   A profile of the work of a primary care physician (from the sources quoted in the text)

Doctor–patient contacts	Minutes per contact	Number per week	Hours per week
Office (consulting room)	10	140	24
Home visits	30	10	5
Hospital work	15	20	5
Phone	—	15	2
Other indirect consultations	—	10	1
Out-of-hours calls	—	5	3
Total	—	200	40

The amount of time spent on each of these is variable. In Britain the mean time for an office consultation is about 7 minutes, in New Zealand and Australia it is 15 minutes and in USA it is 20 minutes. For home visits the time will depend on distances travelled, but 15–30 minutes is the quoted average. For hospital work it depends whether the physician is carrying out a lengthy procedure or a follow-up round, but 10–15 minutes per patient is a generous average. The 200 contacts represent a 40-hour week, but there is a range from over 60 hours quoted in New Zealand to less than 30 hours in some British practices.

To this profile of work have to be added possible extra professional tasks including: postgraduate exercises, such as clinical meetings, seminars, lecture-discussions; committee and administrative work; teaching and research. Our typical primary physician may therefore be working a 45–50-hour week.

TEMPORAL TRENDS

Work patterns in primary care are not static. In Britain there are data on the trends of consultation (doctor–patient contacts) rates extending back sometimes over 30 years. These have been collected in the Royal College of General Practitioners' publication *Trends in General Practice* (Fry, 1977). There are data from twelve practices that have kept regular and continuing records and there is the data from two national morbidity surveys carried out during 1955–6 and 1970–1 involving around one hundred practitioners in each survey. These show a fall in consulting rates. Home visiting rates have decreased by 60% and office consulting rates by 20%.

I have kept records of all face-to-face consultations in my practice since 1947. My work as measured by consultations per person (patient) per year has halved during this period (Figure 5.1). Most of the reductions were in home visiting, but appreciable falls also occurred in office consultations.

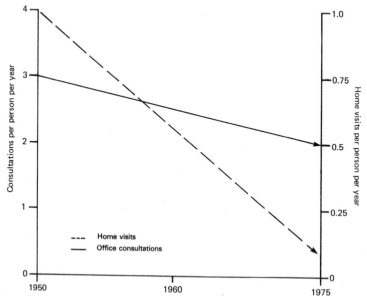

Figure 5.1   Trends in work patterns in a general practice from 1947 to 1976.

Consulting rates are measured as total numbers of annual consultations divided by the population at risk. Such annual consulting rates per person are more accurate representations of work patterns than simple statements of numbers of consultations. Such rates are difficult to calculate when the population at risk is unknown or uncertain. It is only possible in a system such as the British NHS where patients register with a general practitioner and he is paid capitation fees only for those who are registered with him. It is important therefore that the numbers are as accurate as possible.

It is probable that the mean annual person-consulting rate in the NHS is around four consultations per person per year. This means that, if in a practice with 2500 registered patients (of whom 65–70% will consult him in a year) a general practitioner has 10 000 face-to-face consultations in a year, there will be a person-consulting rate of 10 000/2500 or four consultations per person per year. Such rates of work or services related to population are important also in planning for future manpower and resource needs (*vide infra*).

Although the mean annual person-consulting rate is four, there are published rates ranging from less than two to more than six. Such a three-fold difference demands explanation. So far the differences cannot be explained by local medical or social morbidity or most other external factors. They appear to be influenced largely by internal features of the practices and their physicians. In the Second National Morbidity Survey (OPCS, 1974) among the participating practices there were some neighbouring practices from the same area with the same local conditions where the consulting rates differed by 2–3 fold.

Two contrary trends in Britain, suggesting increasing workloads in general practice have been the prescribing rates by general practitioners and market research surveys for pharmaceutical companies. Medication can be obtained under the NHS with a prescription signed by a general practitioner. The Department of Health and Social Security in its annual reports gives the annual prescription rate per person. That is the numbers of prescriptions issued divided by the population. This has shown an increase from five annual prescriptions in the 1950s to over six prescriptions in 1975. Since the annual face-to-face consulting rate is four, a prescribing rate of six must mean that at least two of the prescriptions were for unseen or indirect consultations and that it has been an

57

increase in the indirect prescriptions that has resulted in the rise in prescribing rates and not any increase in face-to-face consultations.

Intercontinental Medical Statistics (IMS) is a market research company that collects information on general practitioner pre-scribing habits by inviting samples of practitioners to keep prospec-tive records of one week's work (IMS, 1977). Among the items recorded are consultations. IMS data show an increase in daily consultations from 32 to 38 over the past decade. Unfortunately there is no information on the definitions of consultations nor of the accuracy and validity of the data.

A PRIMARY MEDICAL MANPOWER MODEL

If we can accept that 10 000 face-to-face consultations is a reasonable volume of work for a primary physician then we can begin to make manpower forecasts for the future. This implies a weekly volume of 200 consultations and a daily volume of 40 consultations for a weekly basic time expenditure of 40 hours or 8 hours a day.

Accepting the 10 000 annual consultations as a fixed target then the future manpower requirements of primary physicians will depend on the annual person consulting rates. Table 5.2 shows the sizes of populations that a primary physician could care for, with a fixed annual total number of 10 000 consultations. It shows also the numbers of primary physicians that would be required for a population of 50 million persons. Thus, with a consulting rate of two consultations per year the primary physician could care for 5000 persons, with a consulting rate of three for 3333, with a con-sulting rate of four for 2500 and with a consulting rate of five for 2000 and with a rate of six for 1667 persons.

For a population of 50 million and a consulting rate of two a health care system will need 10 000 primary physicians and for a consulting rate of six, 30 000 physicians. It now requires a capital expenditure of £1 million ($2 million) to train, pay, support and pension each primary physician in the British NHS and the differ-ence of £20 000 million ($40 000 million) between the costs of these two numbers of physicians is a huge sum that has to be considered most carefully.

Some primary physicians are able to provide apparently good care working at a rate of two annual person-consultations and others work at a rate of six providing care with similar outcome. In planning the intended work rates must be taken into account.

Table 5.2 Model of patients per primary physician for total annual consultations of 10 000

Consulting rates per person per year	Patients per physician for total annual consultations of 10 000	Numbers of primary physicians for a population of 50 million
× 2	5000	10 000
× 3	3333	15 000
× 4	2500	20 000
× 5	2000	25 000
× 6	1667	30 000

QUALITY

Quality of care is as elusive as a mirage and more so in primary care than in other medical fields. Major problems are those of definition and measurement, but there also is the problem of who does the measuring and assessing. Should we be more interested in the subjective satisfactions of consumers on the ways in which they are cared for and treated, or should we place more reliance in planning on the objective measurements of the structure, process and outcome of care as recorded by medical economists and scientists?

Further problems in primary care are that the nature of the conditions is such that many are relatively benign, self-limiting and self-resolving, for which the end points of active treatment may be indistinguishable from those in whom no treatment has been given.

Nevertheless, in spite of such problems attempts must be made to define quality, to measure it, to create models of excellence to be followed, and to provide incentives, facilities and resources by which high quality of care may be achieved.

INFLUENCES

The volume and patterns of work are influenced by many and various factors. These must be recognized, examined and changed, perhaps, if future methods are to be improved.

Customs and habits

Many of the customs and habits of utilizing medical services are ingrained in traditions and beliefs. These may be familial, communal, regional or national. They may be based on cultural, religious or other beliefs. In Chapter 4, the variations in consulting patterns have been noted and there is urgent need to study and understand why patients utilize health services in the ways that they do and also to assess the real benefits of the services provided.

Customs and habits are developed and acquired also by the medical profession and individual habits are built up by physicians. Every physician has his (or her) own habits of diagnosis, investigation and treatment. The usefulness or non-usefulness of current medical habits and customs must be evaluated. Many may be not only useless but potentially dangerous and wasteful.

Expectations

Never before have public and professional expectations of medical care been greater. They now exceed reality. The true scope of medicine is still limited. One effect of positive health education and liberal medical information on the media has been the building up of an over-expectant and over-demanding public. It is time now to develop a more honest form of negative health education of the public and to point out the limitations of what medicine and physicians can achieve and to concentrate more on the responsibilities of the individual in his own health maintenance and self-care.

Money incentives

In many health systems medical care is still a business and the physicians are concerned in selling their skills and services. This is notable where fees-for-services are the methods of remuneration. Thus, the more services that are provided and the more expensive they are, the greater will be the physician's income. This does not happen in systems where payment of physicians is by capitation fees or by salary, the physician's income remains the same whether the patient is sick or well, and whatever the services provided.

These fee-incentives may be one explanation for the disproportionate popularity of well-patient care in the USA and Canada, with frequent check-ups, screening and tests. It may be an explanation for the rates of surgical operations – such as hysterectomy, circumcision, tonsillectomy, cholecystectomy and appendicectomy – which are three-fold higher in North America than in Britain (Bunker, Barnes and Mosteller, 1972).

Morbidity and poverty

Even in welfare societies such as Britain and Sweden there are regional differences in morbidity and mortality rates and in the extent of social pathologies between the different social classes. Such differences influence work demands and needs less than expected. In the British Morbidity Surveys there were no good correlations between low social class areas and high work rates (OPCS, 1974).

Practice organization

A major influence on work volume has been the evolution of the primary care team where work can be shared between physician, home nurse, public health nurse, social worker and medical secretary. The solo single-handed do-it-all himself physician now is an anachronism and wastes his training and his talents. Much of the old traditional physician work can be delegated to, and shared with, his nursing and other colleagues.

Disincentives

Mention has to be made of the use of disincentives and barriers to the use of medical services. High fees, inaccessible units, long waits and delays, non-sympathetic care, and unsafe and unpleasant treatment may all act as barriers to the public.

Education, motivations and effectiveness of the physician

A primary physician who is specially trained and educated for the special field of primary care should use his time and resources better than one who is trained as a would-be but failed hospital specialist, or specialoid. His training should help him to understand the challenges, the nature, the diseases, the methods and the problems of primary care. He will be able to use his resources better and work well with his para-medical colleagues.

61

If he is given also the simple and relatively inexpensive resources needed then he will provide economic, effective and efficient care satisfying to himself and to his patients.

FUTURE IMPLICATIONS

'Work' is a flexible medical commodity. A remarkable similarity exists among primary physicians in developed countries of an annual volume of 10 000 consultations, that is approximately 200 per week, 40 per day with a mean weekly work time of 40 hours per physician. Yet there are large differences influenced by habits of individual physicians. Whilst some physicians, and I am one, can provide for 5000 care of a sound and reasonable quality and others find that caring for 1500 patients is a strain, then it is imperative that we try to discover the reasons for these differences.

Providing that the primary physician is trained for his special roles and tasks; providing that he is sufficiently curious to carry out continuing self-assessment and simple research on his practice to test what is useful and useless in his work; providing that he adopts simple time-saving and effective methods of care; providing that he is supported by a collaborative and well-trained team of nursing, social work and secretarial colleagues with whom he can share his work; providing that he has ready access to diagnostic and therapeutic facilities; providing that he is encouraged by suitable incentives and leadership to achieve good quality care and avoid waste of resources and time; and providing that he has good relations and mutual understanding with his patients and with his colleagues then, with these provisos, I see no reason why we should not be aiming for one primary physician to 3000, 4000 or even 5000 patients.

References

American Medical Association (1976). *Profile of Medical Practice* (Chicago: AMA)
Baker, A. S. *et al.* (1976). *Mo. Med.*, **64**, 213
Bunker, J. P., Barnes, B. A. and Mosteller, F. (eds.) (1977). *Costs, Risks and Benefits of Surgery* (New York: Oxford University Press)
Fry, J. (1969). *Medicine in Three Societies* (Lancaster: MTP Press Limited)
Fry, J. (ed.) (1977). *Trends in General Practice* (London: Royal College of General Practitioners)
Intercontinental Medical Statistics (1977). Personal communication.

Kohn, R. and White, K. L. (1976). *Health Care* (New York and London: Oxford University Press)

Lough, J. D. (1967). *N. Z. Med. J.*, **66**, Supplement

Marsh, G. N., Wallace, R. B. and Whewell, J. (1976). *Br. Med. J.*, **1**, 1321

Office of Population Censuses and Surveys (1974). *Statistics from General Medical Practice, Second National Morbidity Survey* (London: HMSO)

Riley, G. J. (1969). *J. Am. Med. Assoc.*, **208**, 2307

Scotton, R. B. and Grounds, A. D. (1969). *Med. J. Aust.*, Supplement No. 1

Wolfe, S. and Badgley, R. F. (1972). *The Family Doctor* (New York: The Milbank Memorial Fund)

6
The Nature and Natural History of Common Diseases

An expectant public has been encouraged by an enthusiastic and optimistic profession to expect and demand a cure for almost every ill and symptom. It becomes difficult to resist the 'do something' demands of the 'gawd sakers' (for God's sake do something doctor!). Nevertheless it is essential that some re-education of both public and profession is carried out as a counterweight, so that we may be able to decide when and where treatment may be unnecessary and un-helpful and to decide when and where the condition should be allowed to follow a natural course and safe outcome. At this time with increasingly potent, and potentially dangerous, drugs and other medical and surgical procedures it is more important than ever to know when not to use them, as it is to know when to use them.

It is necessary to learn and to understand the nature and the natural history, course and outcome of the common diseases if we are to have sound baselines with which the advantages of modern medicine can be measured and compared. It is in the field of primary care that the nature and natural history can best be studied and learnt, for the reasons and examples that follow. It is in primary care that the opportunities for further study and research exist.

There are general practices in Britain and other societies where the same practice has provided primary health care for the same community for over one hundred years, by successive generations of primary family physicians, and whose experience and know-ledge of the course and outcome of diseases as they affected their patients would provide unique pictures of natural history, had reasonably accurate, accessible and analysable records have been kept. Unfortunately this has not been the case. Records, knowledge and experience of individuals, families and communities have usually followed the physician into retirement or into the grave and have been lost at one stroke.

What I have done, or tried to do, is to keep simple records in an accessible and analysable form in my own practice for over 30 years and the observations that follow are based on these records.

ON THE NATURE OF DISEASE

Let us be honest and humble. Let us accept and acknowledge the huge limitations and gaps in our knowledge of the nature of many of the common diseases. We do not know what causes rheumatism and its syndromes; we do not know the causes of cancer; we do not know why some individuals suffer from migraine, from peptic ulcers, from asthma or from colitis. We may be defining the risk factors of coronary artery disease and chronic bronchitis, but we are no closer to understanding the causes. We know little about the most common forms of high blood pressure or essential hypertension. We know less than little about the true nature and causes of the common respiratory infections, about the common psychiatric and behavioural disorders, and about the common skin disorders. This list could be extended on and on.

Our lack of knowledge of the causation, nature and course of these common disorders means that we cannot base our nomenclature, management and treatment of them on any sound specific foundations. There is much more research to be done, but in the meantime we have to do what we can to help those in need, using the knowledge that we have.

TRUE SPECTRUM OF DISEASE

The benefits of specialization are that the specialist becomes more experienced with, and knows more and more about, a narrower and smaller part of the whole. The defects of specialization are the dangers of losing a sense of perspective and acknowledging that the specialist often sees but a small part of the true spectrum of a disease or syndrome. In conditions such as high blood pressure, asthma,

66

migraine, rheumatoid arthritis, coronary artery disease, strokes, backache, diabetes and similar disorders, the hospital specialist sees a small tip of a clinical iceberg; the primary physician sees a much greater proportion but some will remain undiagnosed or will be self-treated.

TRUE PERSPECTIVE OF DISEASE

As well as seeing only part of the clinical whole of a disorder the specialist will be handicapped in other ways, and so will the students that he teaches and the junior doctors (residents) and nurses who work in hospital.

The patients and their problems who are referred to and reach specialists and hospitals are a highly selected collection. They do not necessarily represent a true picture of the disease, disorder or syndrome. In the confines of a clinic or a hospital, people with diseases are in an unnatural situation. They are akin to animals in a zoo, captive and confined and unable to be seen in their natural state or habitat. Whereas in the community, the place of primary care, they are as in the jungle, living in their own homes and environment. It is difficult, if not impossible, for the hospital specialist to know what goes on in the patient's life and circumstances outside the hospital's walls. It is the essence of good primary care to know much about the families, the homes, the occupations and the living environment of his local practice community.

There is another difference. The hospital or specialist experience of, and contact with, a typical person is but with two or three incidents in a lifetime. A feature of primary care is long-term and continuing care and between patient and doctor. It is as though the hospital or specialist episode is but an instant snapshot of a person with a disease at that particular moment of time, whereas the features of primary care provide a life-long running movie film.

To give an illustration of the numerical differences in the clinical experiences between a general practitioner and consultants in his local district hospital, Table 6.1 shows the numbers of patients with certain common diseases that one average general practitioner with a practice of 2500 persons may see in one year and the numbers that consultants in various specialties may see in their hospital work in a year in the British NHS.

Table 6.1 Numbers of patients seen annually by a general practitioner and a hospital consultant in the British NHS (from Fry, 1977a, 1977b)

Condition	General practitioner (per 2500)	Hospital consultant (per 250 000)
Respiratory		
Upper respiratory infections	600	? nil
Pneumonia and bronchitis	50	100
Asthma	30	50
Enlarged tonsils and adenoids for removal	6	250
Cardio-vascular		
Myocardial infarction	8	125
High blood pressure	5 (new)	75 (new)
	30 (continuing)	200 (continuing)
Varicose veins	20	75
Cancers		
Lung	3	50
Breast	1	25
Large bowel	2	30
Alimentary		
Peptic ulcers	25	60
Acute appendicitis	5	100
Hernia	7	150
Haemorrhoids	10	100
Gall bladder	2	30
Others		
Uterine fibroids	3	100
Rheumatoid arthritis	10	200
Diabetes	1 (new)	40 (new)
	10 (continuing)	250 (continuing)
Strokes	5	120
Anxiety/Depression	250	100

NATURAL HISTORY: THE TEMPORAL DIMENSION

Analysis of data of incidence, prevalence and outcome of patients in my practice with the more common diseases and adding to this the results from the OPCS Morbidity Survey (1974), five patterns of natural history are apparent. These patterns relate to diseases that are likely to go on for some years and not to short-lived disorders where the outcomes are obvious (Figure 6.1).

Type 1: 'Once and Always' These disorders once they arise will persist and continue for as long as the patient lives, although some

68

of their effects can be relieved. Examples of these are congenital disorders such as mongolism, phenylketonuria and cystic fibrosis. Diabetes and hypothyroidism, once they have developed will persist, so will hemiplegia and similar disorders.

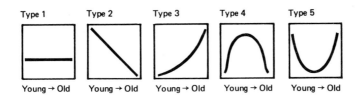

Figure 6.1   Five patterns of natural history of disease.

Type 2: 'Disorders that children outgrow'   Many children develop disorders which they outgrow naturally and spontaneously. An example is the catarrhal child syndrome (Fry, 1961), which includes, coughs, colds, earache, sore throat and wheezy chest. These conditions are all most prevalent between 4 and 8 years and after 8 they become less and less frequent. Other conditions that improve are umbilical herniae, strawberry naevi, knock-knees, bow-legs and non-retractible foreskins.

Type 3: 'Disorders of ageing'   As we live longer so we are more likely to suffer from disorders of ageing and degeneration. Thus their prevalence will increase and so will their severity, with time. Examples are, osteoarthritis, coronary artery disease, high blood pressure, cancers, strokes, chronic bronchitis, cataracts and deafness.

Type 4: 'Come and go'   This is a pattern where the onset is generally in early or mid-adult life; there follows a period of clinical activity for 10–20 years, often in a periodic or intermittent manner; and then symptoms tend to diminish and finally to disappear (Fry, 1974). This course occurs in asthma, migraine, acute backache, hay fever, duodenal ulcer, anxiety-depression and urinary tract infections.

Type 5: 'Young and old'   Then there are syndromes, or collections of symptoms and signs, that are most prevalent in the young and the old, with a low prevalence in the age-periods between (Fry, 1966). The conditions that fit this pattern are acute wheezy chest, constipation, herniae and hydrocoeles.

IMPLICATIONS

There is much that is unique in the nature of the experience with disease and its management in primary care. It provides a fuller picture and a better understanding of the whole disease and not just one specialist part of it. It offers opportunities to study the long-term course and outcome.

Particularly, it is important to apply the lessons of the patterns of natural history. It is wrong to treat over-energetically conditions that have a strong likelihood of improving naturally. This applies with special force to children's disorders such as the common respiratory infections. Care and discrimination must be applied to wholesale removal of tonsils and adenoids and to over-ready use of antibiotics. Likewise, the type 4 pattern of 'come and go' should be appreciated and optimism and encouragement are justifiable in the management of conditions in this group.

Over-enthusiasm must also be tempered with the progressive disorders of ageing. Relieve and comfort by all means, but beware of the impossible in attempting 'cures' by dangerous means.

References

Fry, J. (1961). *The Catarrhal Child* (London: Butterworth)

Fry, J. (1966). *Profiles of Disease* (Edinburgh: E. and S. Livingstone)

Fry, J. (1974). *Common Diseases* (Lancaster: MTP Press Limited)

Fry, J. (1977a). *Update*, **15**, 829

Fry, J. (1977b). *J. R. Coll. Gen. Practit.*, **27**, 9

Office of Population Censuses and Surveys (OPCS) (1974). *Second National Morbidity Survey* (London: HMSO)

7
Cure and Care

UNNECESSARY DILEMMAS

Over the past few years antagonisms have arisen within medical education, research and service over some fundamental aspects of the nature and objectives of medical practice. The line-up has been on a number of fronts (Table 7.1) but broadly they are those that can be grouped under the more vague, comfortable and warm caring roles and those grouped under the more specific, sharp and coldly scientific curing roles.

Table 7.1   The cure and care dilemma

Cure	vs	Care
Science		Art
Clinical		Pastoral
Biological		Behavioural and social
Physical		Emotional
Disease		Person
Body		Soul
Hospital		Community
First class		Second class

It is as though cure and care have become polarized attracting their own sets of features and values. In some ways this has been true and it is noticeable that there has been an emphasis, some would say an over-emphasis, on scientific biological and clinical aspects of diseases in medical schools and hospitals, where young medical men and women in training have been brought up to believe that this work and research is first-class and best. There has been a definite tendency for medical teachers and researchers to view 'care' in the community as a soft option for those who have been unable to achieve a career in the hard cold scientific climate of medicine within the hospital specialties. To quote the late Lord Moran's views stated in evidence to the Royal Commission on Medical Education in 1965, he believed that those in primary care had 'fallen off the (medical) ladder' and were, by implication, medicine's second-class citizens.

GOOD CARE

Such polarizations, views and posturings are quite unrealistic and even crazy. There can be no divisions over cure and care in the management of our patients. It is not possible to do one without involving the other. It is as wrong to be over-caring as to be over-curing and as wrong to under-care as to under-cure. The good practice of medicine in all fields and specialties demands a holism that involves a good mix of scientific and technological skills and humane understanding of the patient as an individual in the context of his, or her, family and society. Good care must be based on caring for the patient as a person.

The good doctor, be he working in primary care in the community or in a most narrow sub-specialty unit in a hidden corner of a hospital, will apply his scientific knowledge, technological skills and clinical experience for his patients with the same feeling and consideration as he would wish them to be applied to himself or his family, were they in the same situation. 'Do unto others what you would have them do to you' is a most appropriate teaching in personal medical care. In this context it is well to consider how much investigation and treatment, not of a pleasant nature, we would wish to undergo when their proven worth is in doubt.

Whilst the treatment of disease may sometimes require an impersonal attitude, with not much emotional involvement, in order to arrive at unbiased and clinical decisions, nevertheless the care of patients must be personal always, with a commitment by the physician to see through the patients' problems. Good care demands very much more from the physician than making a diagnosis, writing a prescription or performing a surgical operation. It challenges us in the more difficult task of achieving personal understanding with, and personal care of, our patients.

MODERN TRENDS

Such laudable acts and actions are made more difficult by trends in modern society and medicine, yet paradoxically they are yearned for more than ever by the people.

The twin summits of modern scientific technology, the atom bomb and sending men on to the moon were made possible by intensive scientific effort and application of modern technological advances. It is understandable that such progress should be sought for in the cure and the care of diseases and medical social problems. Why, reasonable people ask, cannot efforts on impersonal acts such as the atom bomb and walking on the moon be focused on helping men and women to live longer healthier lives? The public is rightly becoming more impatient and more expectant of medical miracles and more demanding of better skills and care.

The atom bomb and the man-on-the-moon philosophy has highlighted the need for specialization in science, in order to achieve advance and progress. So in medicine the emphasis on specialization has been building up for the past 50 years or more. It is reasonable for the man in the street to assume that specialists are the best physicians to consult in times of sickness. The specialization cult has developed, encouraged by the medical profession and supported with enthusiasm by the public.

Neither seem to have appreciated the true nature of disease and its problems (Chapters 3 and 6) and that at the primary and secondary levels of disease care there still is a desperate need to have good generalists who can make proper assessments of the possible needs for sub-specialist referrals and to carry out those tasks and roles still best done by generalists.

Another trend linked partly to increasing specialization and over-complexity of techniques of care has been the evolution of teams and teamwork. Within specialties there has developed in-speciality sub-specialization with splintering of tasks. Teams are formed to support specialists and the care of the individual patient is shared not just between doctors and nurses but between specialist physicians and nurses and also shared with other technicians and auxiliaries. All this has led to escalating costs of care but more important it has made personal care of the patient increasingly difficult, if not impossible. It has caused crises of anxiety and uncertainty among patients and it may have added to iatrogenic risks.

There is a great need for each patient to have a personal professional protector to take him by the hand and to guide him safely through the hidden, and not so hidden, hazards of the medical jungle. There is need for a primary physician to maintain a continuing responsibility as the personal medical adviser, to assess and to decide on the care needed, to refer to other specialists and to work with them as an equal in providing what is necessary and to ensure that it is well done in a safe and least distressing manner.

The pendulum is swinging away from over-expectancy of specialization and super-specialization in medicine, back towards the realization that it is false logic and false economy to over-rely on specialists and that in all systems a personal primary physician is essential, being someone to initiate care, see it through and halt it at the appropriate time.

To achieve 'cures' modern medical technologies have to be centralized at special units but the 'care' given always must be of a personal nature related to the needs of each individual patient.

WHAT DO WE SEEK OF MEDICAL CARE?

Inevitably there are different groups concerned in care; the patient, the physician and the providers. In general all these seek similar objectives; the best possible care for all at the most economic cost. In detail however the three groups have differing priorities.

The patient will place high priority on a personal and humane approach with an understanding of his or her special individual problems. The care to be provided by a well-trained professional who has the skills and experience to carry out what is necessary. Although the criteria of success is a satisfactory outcome of the problems, 'tender loving care with a good bedside manner' are high priorities.

The physician's first priority must be to cure his patient whenever and wherever possible; failing this to provide appropriate relief and comfort. There are in addition other professional 'wants'. Trained as a biological scientist in modern medical methods he seeks to use his skills. He needs good diagnostic and therapeutic resources by which to apply his skills. He seeks freedom from wants for his patient and himself—that is his patients should not be restricted by shortages of funds to pay for care—and he seeks reasonable and adequate financial rewards for his professional services. Ideally, financial transactions should not be part of medical care, but some believe that there are advantages in patients paying for at least a part of the medical bill.

He seeks co-operation and collaboration from his patients. He wants them to fit into his pattern of organization and he would like them to be educated and informed enough to participate in their own preventive and therapeutic activities. Such collaboration requires public education in the use of local health services and in the process of medical communication. It is a part of health education that has been neglected. The teaching of the simple rules of self-health and of the rules of the use of health care resources must be high priorities in all systems.

The providers may be a government responsible for a national health service, a public facility or a private insurance enterprise, but whoever they are they are concerned with similar objectives. They seek to make possible good care for all those for whom they are responsible. They want this care to be effective, efficient and economic. They want this to be satisfactory to consumers and satisfying to the professional. To achieve all this there has to be some system of organization and administration that includes quality and quantity controls and assessments.

The correct compromise mixture of all these 'wants' and 'needs' has to be evolved by every health care system in relation to its own historical development, its own political, cultural and social beliefs, to its own economic, physical and manpower resources, and to its own geographical and climatic features.

FACTORS IN CURE AND CARE

For the best results in achieving cure and care, attention must be paid to a knowledge of the following eight factors. This applies to all levels of care, to specialist and sub-specialist care in hospitals just as much as in primary care.

1 The patient as an individual

The patient is not a lump of cold flesh bringing clear and defined diseases to be managed according to the book. Each patient has his (or her) own behavioural and social background to be considered and also his own package of past clinical and disease experience. Each person reacts in an individual manner to medical, social, or personal problems. The manner of reaction will determine the modes of presentation, the degrees of tolerance and the extent of anxiety.

Each consultation should include such questions as: why has this particular patient consulted me at this time? why does he present his symptoms in the ways that he has? what sort of person is he and how is he likely to react to treatment? what does he expect of the consultation? It is far easier to have the answers in the setting of primary personal care where continuity enables the physician to know his patient well over years of regular contact and where each consultation is part of a long-term follow-up and not a new meeting.

2 The family unit

Individuals are members of a family unit or group. The family is the basic social unit where first-level health care is practised (see Chapter 4). Knowledge of how an individual fits and fares in his own family is important in providing care. Does he have a family? What does his family compromise? How restricted or how extended is it? How good are interpersonal relations within his family? What is the family history in regard to disease, patterns of consultation, and coping and self-help?

3 Social environment

Knowledge of the individual's social environment extends widely. Of relevance and importance are his occupation, its hazards, satisfactions and dissatisfactions. Conditions of housing and social amenities are important and they can be known only by home visiting. Quite apart from the physical state of the house and its contents, a home visit provides information on housekeeping and managerial abilities, on hygienic levels and on degrees of overcrowding.

Poverty and wealth are personal, community and national characteristics, and they influence levels of health and prevalence of disease most profoundly.

4 Disease

In Chapter 5 the nature of disease at the primary care level was discussed. A knowledge of the natural history, course and outcome of the common diseases is essential for sound care.

5 Management

From a knowledge of disease it is possible to begin to make decisions on:

What is normal or a normal abnormality that requires no treatment.

What is tolerable, as far as the individual patient is concerned. This applies to relief rather than to cure. Tolerance is a very individual matter and the physician has to make a decision based on his knowledge of his patient.

What is curable. Heroic and vain attempts at cure are to be deplored, particularly if the cure is more grievous to bear than the disease.

What is preventable. Whilst prevention is a laudable objective, it must again be stated honestly that in few of the common diseases have preventive measures been successful. Whilst the benefits of ceasing to smoke, to take regular exercise and to eat and drink in moderation are accepted they are difficult to achieve. The benefits of diets, varied pills and check-ups are unproven (see page 24).

6 Drug and other therapies

There are fads and fashions in drug and other therapies. Any physician who has been in practice for 10 years or more can recall already how certain drugs have been introduced, have reached high levels of popularity, have caused serious, but few, side effects, have then become less popular and eventually have reached a more balanced level of usefulness.

It is unsafe to be the first or the last to use a drug or other therapy. One can be too early and unaware of its place, actions and side-effects, or too late when others have given it up because of its dangers or non-success.

All that we do therapeutically must be assessed critically. Ideally, clinical trials are necessary and there is no doubt that the general practitioner is uniquely placed to investigate those areas of medicine which have become his exclusive domain (Murphy, 1977). Whilst such trials may not be easy at the single practitioner or practice level, nevertheless it is possible to ask ourselves 'is this treatment really necessary?' whenever we are motivated to write a prescription or to carry out a procedure.

7 Local facilities

The primary physician has to be expert in becoming familiar with local health, medical and social facilities and resources. He has to know what is available, what is useful, who is good, who is dangerous. Even more he has to learn how to manipulate and fit local facilities (or more distant ones) for the good of his patients. He has to try to match the right specialist for his patient's needs. No two surgeons, for example, are of the same calibre, or the same personality. No two psychiatrists are the same and it may be difficult, sometimes, to get the correct mix of patient and specialist. The role of the personal primary physician must be to be constantly available as the arbiter and translator of the specialist's advice and views. It should not be uncommon for the personal physician not to agree with a specialist and with his long knowledge of his patient he may be in a better position to decide what should, or should not, be carried out diagnostically or therapeutically. The role of the primary personal physician is that of a puppet-master with specialists as his puppets. The puppets will move only when the master moves the strings. This applies also to the use of social services and of the work of the primary care team. There has to be a personal physician who can assume long-term responsibilities as his patients' ultimate adviser, physician, philosopher and friend.

8 Self-knowledge and self-awareness

A most difficult piece of knowledge is knowing oneself as a physician. How much or how little should we do? What motivations and incentives lead us to do what we do? How does our care compare with that of others?

In theory, self-audit and a self-profile or critique, should help to answer these questions, but the methods of audit are uncertain and their wide-scale applications have not been successful in primary care. This does not mean that their objectives should not be pursued.

IMPLICATIONS

There must be no dilemmas of care versus cure. The two are inseparable. All who seek to cure must also care. We have to combine measurements of cure with the unmeasurable, but well appreciated, attributes of care. The good physician must be that one who will always combine his successful cures with kindly, humane and understanding care and who will accept also his social and public responsibilities and endeavour to persuade his patients to do likewise.

Reference

Murphy, J. E. (1977). *Clinical Trials in General Practice* in F. N. Johnson and S. Johnson (eds.), *Clinical Trials*, pp. 176–87 (Oxford: Blackwell Scientific Publications Limited)

Further reading

Cochrane, A. L. (1971). *Effectiveness and Efficiency* (London: Nuffield Provincial Hospitals Trust)

Cooper, M. H. (1975). *Rationing Health Care* (London: Croom Helm)

Dubos, R. (1960). *Mirage of Health* (London: George Allen and Unwin)

Fuchs, V. R. (1974). *Who Shall Live?* (New York: Basic Books)

Godber, G. E. (1975). *Change in Medicine* (London: Nuffield Provincial Hospitals Trust)

Knowles, J. H. (1977). Doing Better and Feeling Worse: Health in the United States, *Daedalus*, **106**, 1

Lalonde, M. (1974). *A New Perspective on the Health of Canadians* (Ottawa: Government of Canada)

McKeown, T. (1976). *The Role of Medicine* (London: Nuffield Provincial Hospitals Trust)

McLachlan, G. (ed.) (1971). *Medical History and Medical Care* (London: Oxford University Press)

McLachlan, G. (ed.) (1976). *A Question of Quality* (London: Oxford University Press)

McLachlan, G. (1977). *Medical Education and Medical Care* (London: Oxford University Press)

Scientific American (1973). *Life and Death and Medicine* (San Francisco: W. H. Freeman and Company)

8
Prescribing

A major therapeutic action that the clinician carries out is the writing out of a prescription for a medicine (medicament). After counselling, medicines are the most frequently used health care resources in contemporary industrial societies. Three out of every four doctor–patient consultations in primary care involve the prescribing of one, and often more than one, medicament. The widespread use of self-medication involving over-the-counter proprietary medicines and the growing interest in old folk remedies also should be appreciated. It is estimated that for every two prescribed medicines there are three non-prescribed taken.

The extent of medicine taking is widespread and increasing both in volume and in cost. In developed societies such as North America and Western Europe each person, man, woman and child, receives on average 5–6 prescribed scripts each year for medicines from primary physicians. The highest quoted rate, of over nine, was in the Netherlands. The cost of each script averages £1.30 ($2.60) in the British NHS and £3 ($6.00) in the USA. This means that a primary physician in the British NHS will prescribe £20 000 ($40 000) of drugs each year for his patients and the same physician in the USA will be responsible for some £30 000 ($60 000) (Silverman and Lee, 1974).

The cost of prescribing by physicians is a major item in health care expenditure. It accounts for 15% of the total cost of health care in the USA, around 10% in the UK and 8% in Canada. In any year 50–60% of all persons will receive one or more prescriptions for a medicine, females more often than males and the educated more than the uneducated.

ADVANCES AND TRENDS

The drug industry is highly competitive and is engaged constantly in research for new and better drugs to help mankind and boost its sales and profits. It has been remarkably successful on both counts. The advances and benefits achieved from the discovery and introduction of antibiotics, psychotropic drugs, corticosteroids, cardiac and anti-hypertensive drugs and many others have been dramatic and beneficial.

The primary physician now has a much wider range of powerful effective drugs than did his father and grandfather. He has much more scope for specific curative therapy with modern drugs than did his forebears who could prescribe only coloured placebo mixtures, that nevertheless were amazingly successful at times. However, with the increased effectiveness and power of modern medicines has come also the power to do harm from dangerous side-effects.

WHY PRESCRIBE?

Why is prescribing and imbibing of medicines by human beings so popular? It is one of the major distinctions between human beings and other mammals. Why is it so universal? It is by no means a special feature only of industrial and developed societies. Given the opportunities and resources, that is money and the medicines, it will be seized upon by all societies. The results of the international study reported by Kohn and White (1976) show that at any time 60% will be consuming medicines, of those 27% will be prescribed and 33% non-prescribed. The highest medication rate was found in Vermont, USA, where 75% of those questioned were taking medicines at the time and the lowest in Yugoslavia, 25%.

The reasons for this human habit must be many and various. A large part of it comes from consumer (patient) demands and expectations. The patient goes to consult his (or her) physician with a problem, a symptom or a diagnosis. He expects something to be done or given, and this is usually a pill or mixture or injection or suppository or balm, depending on local customs.

Medicine still is a mystical art, supported by science. The physician still has a high social status and is held in fear and awe. He has the knowledge and power to help with the unknown, illness and sickness. He is consulted in the hope and the expectation that he will do something to cure or relieve. He is expected to be an activist doer, rather than a non-doer.

The nature of disease and problems in primary care (Chapters 3 and 6) is such that many (65%) are minor, some (20%) are chronic and a few (15%) are acute and major. It is also a fact that many of the minor and chronic conditions will quickly or slowly improve naturally. Dramatic and instant medicinal cures are exceptions. As a rough guide it may be that 20% of primary care conditions are curable quickly and dramatically, 70% are relievable, but that in 100% the physician should try to comfort his patient.

Another reason for high prescribing is that it is far quicker and easier for the physician to prescribe than not to. If he does not, he will have to spend time and effort in explanations and in convincing the patient that no medication is required. The result of such negative efforts is a dissatisfied patient, who will often consult another prescribing physician.

Then, in free-enterprise societies there is the persuasive influence of the drug industry, which has to sell competitively in order to exist, to produce, to research and to develop. Most of its selling efforts and advertising are aimed at the primary physician and the public. Silverman and Lee (1974) show that the drug industry now has the highest rate of advertising expenditure, over 10% of the sale income, of any industry in the USA.

Missing from the whole exercise of prescribing and use of drugs are any reliable facts on the efficacy of the many drugs used. There is a great difference between diseases of primary care and the drugs used, and the diseases and therapies of specialist practice. Controlled trials have been undertaken on few drugs used in primary care and not under the special conditions of primary care. There is a need to discover through controlled clinical trials how best to use psychotropic drugs, antibiotics, and other groups of drugs for the common disorders (Johnson and Johnson, 1977).

Until we know more about what is being prescribed, why and with what effects, we should adopt a highly self-critical attitude to whatever we prescribe and ask ourselves whether the prescription is really necessary, whether the particular drug prescribed is the best or can a safer and cheaper one be used?

83

WHAT IS PRESCRIBED?

There is a piecemeal collection of reports on the content of prescriptions given by physicians and of over-the-counter non-prescribed medicines. The data is presented in various forms using different classifications. The general findings are that whilst the same types of problems and diseases are being managed in primary care everywhere, local customs, habits and attitudes influence the patterns of prescribing and account for the differences.

The most comprehensive and extensive data is from the British

Table 8.1   Prescriptions for drugs in England during 1974: population, 46 million; general practitioners, 20 000; prescriptions, 275 million (from DHSS, 1977)

Therapeutic group	Number of prescriptions (in millions)	Per cent
Nervous system		
Tranquillizers	20	
Analgesics	18	
Hypnotics	17	
Anti-depressants	8	
Total	74	28
Antibiotics		
Penicillins	18	
Tetracyclines	10	
Total	38	15
Cardio-vascular system		
Diuretics	11	
Heart preparations	7	
Anti-hypertensives	6	
Total	30	11
Lower respiratory tract		
Cough medicines	17	
Anti-spasmodics	8	
Total	27	10
Alimentary system		
Antacids	9	
Laxatives	7	
Sedatives and bitters	4	
Total	20	8
Skin		
Corticosteroids	10	
Total	18	7

National Health Service. Table 8.1 shows the volume of prescriptions for various groups of preparations in England with a population of 46 million and with some 20 000 general practitioners.

In a study of 100 000 prescriptions from a population of 40 000 in England in a year, Skegg *et al.* (1977) found that 17% of the prescriptions were for psychotropic drugs, 14% for antibiotics, 12% for cardiovascular system, 10% for respiratory system, 10% for analgesics and 6% each for skin preparations and for alimentary system drugs.

Parish (1976) found the top ten preparations in a study in the UK to be, in order, cough mixtures, analgesics, tranquillizers, penicillins, barbiturates, tetracyclines, corticosteroid skin preparations, bronchial antispasmodics, antacids and rheumatic preparations.

The international study by Kohn and White (1976) quotes findings in percentages of persons taking prescribed and non-prescribed drugs at any time and Table 8.2 shows these. Of prescribed drugs in adults, heart preparations, analgesics and vitamins were the most frequently taken groups of drugs and in children, vitamins (in 38%) and cough mixtures. Of non-prescribed drugs and analgesics, vitamins and cough medicines were the most frequently taken.

Table 8.2 Percentages of persons taking prescribed and non-prescribed medicines (from Kohn and White, 1976)

Therapeutic group	*% Prescribed*		*% Non-prescribed*	
	Adults	*Children*	*Adults*	*Children*
Vitamins	11	38	15	31
Analgesics .	12	—	43	24
Cough medicines	—	20	12	17
Skin preparations	—	—	11	13
Laxatives	7	—	11	4
Heart preparations	14	—	—	—
Tranquillizers	9	—	—	—
Sleeping-pills	5	—	—	—
All		27		33

VARIATIONS IN PRESCRIBING PATTERNS

Assuming that in primary care in developed industrial societies the morbidity is similar, it is extraordinary how the volume and content of prescriptions differ. The differences occur at all levels, internationally, regionally, locally and within the same practice. In fact no two physicians will have the same prescribing profiles.

In the UK there is a 20% regional difference in volume of prescribing between the highest in North-west England (in Merseyside) and the lowest in the South-west (Oxford). There are even greater differences in the different volumes of therapeutic groups. Dunlop and Inch (1972) noted a six-fold difference in prescribing tonics between Sweden and the UK, being much higher in Sweden. Gamma globulin was used ten times more in Sweden than in the UK. The prescribing of phenylbutazone was four times greater in Switzerland than in neighbouring France. In France cholagogues are popular and used forty times more frequently than in the UK; likewise French physicians favour calcium supplements, prescriptions for lactobacillus and administration of medicines as supposi-

Table 8.3 Use of prescribed medicines in various countries (from Kohn and White, 1976)

Therapeutic group	Percentage of people		
	Median	Highest	Lowest
Children			
Vitamins	38	57 (Helsinki)	10 (Canada)
Cough medicines	20	30 (Liverpool and Yugoslavia)	14 (USA and Canada)
Adults			
Heart preparations	14	20 (Helsinki)	3 (Canada)
Analgesics	14	26 (Yugoslavia)	8 (Canada)
Vitamins	11	20 (Poland)	6 (Yugoslavia)
Tranquillizers	9	14 (Buenos Aires)	6 (Canada)
Sleeping-pills	5	8 (Liverpool)	4 (Canada)
Laxatives	7	11 (Buenos Aires)	5 (Helsinki)
All	27	34 (USA and Canada)	16 (Yugoslavia and Poland)

tories. Spa therapy has become extinct in the UK. It is still very popular in France, Germany, Switzerland, Eastern Europe and the USSR. Acupuncture is a Chinese all-purpose remedy.

More specifically the ranges of prescribed and non-prescribed drugs found by Kohn and White (1976) are notable (Tables 8.3 and 8.4). Some striking patterns are evident. Vitamins are popular in Helsinki, analgesics in Yugoslavia and laxatives in Liverpool. No obvious explanations are evident.

Table 8.4   Use of non-prescribed drugs in various countries (from Kohn and White, 1976)

Therapeutic group	Percentage of people		
	Median	Highest	Lowest
Children			
Vitamins	31	59 (Helsinki)	8 (Buenos Aires)
Analgesics	24	61 (Yugoslavia)	7 (Helsinki)
Cough medicines	17	30 (Poland)	12 (Canada)
Skin preparations	13	22 (Liverpool)	5 (Buenos Aires)
Laxatives	4	8 (Liverpool)	1 (Helsinki)
Adults			
Vitamins	15	29 (Helsinki)	2 (Yugoslavia)
Analgesics	43	69 (Yugoslavia)	33 (Helsinki)
Cough medicines	12	16 (Helsinki)	8 (Buenos Aires)
Skin preparations	11	18 (Canada)	3 (Buenos Aires)
Laxatives	11	16 (Liverpool)	2 (Yugoslavia)
All	33	40 (USA and Canada)	10 (Yugoslavia and Poland)

The rate of use of medicines in the twelve areas reported by Kohn and White (1976) are shown in Table 8.5. Here the three-fold difference between the highest use in north-west Vermont, USA (74% of persons taking prescribed or non-prescribed drugs) and the

87

Table 8.5 Percentages of the population using prescribed and non-prescribed medicines in various parts of the world (from Kohn and White, 1976)

	Canada				USA		South America	West Europe		East Europe			All
	GP	SA	FR	JE	NV	BE	BA	LL	HE	LO	BT	RT	
Prescribed medicines	27	30	26	27	34	33	30	25	28	19	16	18	27
Non-prescribed medicines	36	38	37	35	40	33	18	32	30	13	10	10	33
Totals	63	68	63	62	74	66	48	57	58	32	26	28	60

GP – Grande Prairie, Alberta
SA – Saskatchewan
FR – Fraser, British Columbia
JE – Jersey, British Columbia

NV – North-west Vermont
BE – Baltimore, Maryland
BA – Buenos Aires
LL – Liverpool

HE – Helsinki
LO – Lodz
BT – Banat, Serbia
RT – Rijeka, Croatia

lowest in Banat, Yugoslavia (26%) is clearly shown. The differences exist both in prescribed and non-prescribed drugs.

The general trends are for high prescribing in the USA and Canada, low rates in Eastern Europe, with Buenos Aires, Liverpool and Helsinki mid-way. It is notable how the rates of use were very similar in the six areas in Canada and the USA, in the two towns in Western Europe, and in the three towns in Eastern Europe.

CHANGES WITH TIME

Nothing remains static in medicine. This applies to prescribing in particular. As an example Table 8.6 shows the numbers of prescriptions in England and Wales for psychotropic drugs from 1965 to 1975. The population did not change much. During this period there were attempts to reduce prescribing of barbiturates and stimulating drugs (amphetamines) and new tranquillizers and antidepressant drugs were introduced with much advertising. The amount of barbiturate hypnotics prescribed by general practitioners was reduced by well over one-half, but this fall was made up by a trebling in amounts of non-barbiturate hypnotics. The prescribing of tranquillizers and anti-depressants doubled and the use of stimulating drugs and appetite suppressants was reduced by one-half.

Table 8.6 Numbers (in millions) of annual prescriptions for psychotropic drugs in England and Wales (from DHSS, 1977)

Therapeutic group	1965	1970	1975	Percentage change
Barbiturate hypnotics	17.2	13.1	7.2	− 60
Non-barbiturate hypnotics	2.9	7.1	10.4	+ 250
Tranquillizers	10.8	17.2	22.0	+ 110
Anti-depressants	3.5	6.4	8.5	+ 140
Stimulating and appetite suppressants	5.3	3.4	2.8	− 50
Totals	39.7	47.2	50.9	+ 30

IMPLICATIONS

Medicine taking is an ingrained human habit. It appears that well over one-half of us are taking some medication, prescribed or non-prescribed. Prescribing rates and costs are going up. Figure 8.1

shows the prescribing rate and cost per prescription in the British NHS (no allowances have been made for inflation). The same trends are evident in all countries, with similar social systems. The numbers of prescriptions have doubled in the USA, trebled in Denmark and quadrupled in the Netherlands over the past 25 years.

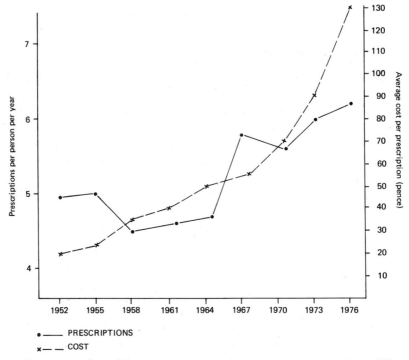

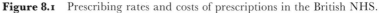

Figure 8.1 Prescribing rates and costs of prescriptions in the British NHS.

The national and international differences in extent of medication are fascinating and the reasons for them should be explored. Why do North Americans swallow three times as many medicines as the East Europeans? There are many hypotheses that come to mind but they need to be tested. More important, what are the effects on health of these different patterns of medication?

The content of prescribed and non-prescribed drugs reflects the morbidity with emotional disorders, infections, respiratory symptoms and degenerative disorders most prevalent. However, when some of the national patterns of prescribing are compared there is confusion and surprise.

From the study of Kohn and White (1976) the surprise is the very high rate of consumption of vitamins. Why do 59% of children and 29% of adults in Helsinki take vitamins, compared with 8% of children in Buenos Aires and 2% of adults in Yugoslavia respectively? Why are more persons in Liverpool and Buenos Aires constipated and taking laxatives than in Helsinki and Yugoslavia? Why are over 60% of children and adults in Yugoslavia taking analgesics? The most likely explanations are those relating to local and national customs and beliefs. Prescribing of medicines and self-medication do not appear to be controlled by any sound scientific rules. It is a huge game with few rules.

Hopes for the future must rest on possible stricter critical examination of the reasons why drugs are prescribed and taken and on much study and assessment of their value and their risks. What is certain is that it is unlikely that the volume of prescribing and taking of medicines will decline very much. What we should achieve is much more sense and sensibility in their use. Prescribe and take medicines if we wish but they should, whenever possible, be safe and cheap, even if they are useless.

References

Department of Health and Social Services (DHSS) (1977). *Personal Social Services Statistics* (London: HMSO)

Dunlop, D. M. and Inch, R. S. (1972). *Br. Med. J.*, **3**, 749

Johnson, F. N. and Johnson, S. (eds.) (1977). *Clinical Trials* (Oxford: Blackwell Scientific Publications Limited)

Kohn, R. and White, K. L. (eds.) (1976). *Health Care* (New York and London: Oxford University Press)

Parish, P., Stimson, G. V., Mapes, R. and Cleary, J. (1976). *J. R. Coll. Gen. Practit.*, **26**, Supplement No. 1

Silverman, M. and Lee, P. R. (1974). *Pills, Profits and Politics* (Berkeley: University of California)

Skegg, D. C. G., Doll, R. and Perry, J. (1977). *Br. Med. J.*, **i**, 1561

9
The Hospital–Primary Care Interface

Hospitals are the most expensive part of any health care system and primary care is the cheapest. Figure 9.1 shows the proportions of money in the British National Health Service (NHS) that are spent on its various parts. The hospital services account for two-thirds of the total annual expenditure, which now is around £6000 million ($20 000 million); primary care services account for 6%, drugs for 8% and dental services for 4%; administration, social services, research, laboratory services and vaccines account for 16% (DHSS, 1977).

Not only are the hospitals most expensive but their share is increasing (Figure 9.1). Over the past 25 years the hospitals' percentage share has gone up by 10% at the expense of all the other parts of the service. One reason for the rising costs of hospitals is simply that they are being used more and more. Figure 9.2 shows the rates at which this has occurred since 1949 in Britain. The greatest increases have been in the use of accident and emergency services, which have doubled.

In 1949, 9% of the population attended hospital accident-emergency departments. Now it is almost 20%. There is no evidence of any similar increase in the rates of major or minor accidents, rather there has been a change in the behaviour patterns of the population. People now attend hospitals for minor injuries and medical conditions more than they did in the past. A possible reason is the lessened availability of British general practitioners.

The proportions of the public admitted to hospital have increased by 70%, from 6.7% in 1949 to 11.1% in 1974. The rates of new

93

referrals (by general practitioners) to hospital specialist out-patient clinics have increased by 20%, from 14% of the population in 1949 to 17% in 1974.

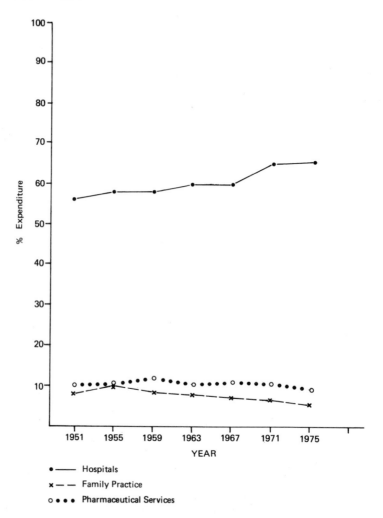

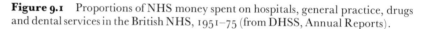

Figure 9.1 Proportions of NHS money spent on hospitals, general practice, drugs and dental services in the British NHS, 1951–75 (from DHSS, Annual Reports).

This suggests that in any year it is theoretically possible that 48% of the population may use the hospital service, but in fact many of the individual users are each using all three departments (accident-

emergency, in-patient and out-patient) and the true rate of utilization is more likely to be around 25%.

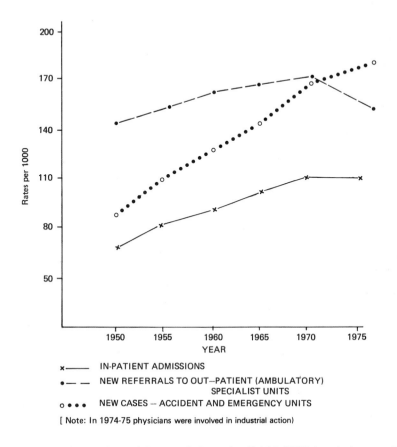

Figure 9.2 Proportions of the population using British NHS hospitals annually
(1949–74) (from DHSS, Annual Reports).

Within the hospitals there has been a great expansion in the work
of the diagnostic departments and they are now also one of the most
expensive. In 1971 it was estimated that the cost of investigatory
(pathological and radiological) services in major acute hospitals in
the British NHS was £3.49 ($6.98) per in-patient week, compared
with £1.83 ($3.66) for drugs and £3.98 ($7.96) for medical salaries
(Ashley, Pasker and Beresford, 1972). The use of these investigatory
departments has more than quadrupled since 1949 (Figure 9.3).

The productivity of the British hospitals has been high in terms of caring for an increasing volume of in-patients, out-patients and accident-emergencies, whilst using fewer (20%) hospital beds and with a 50% shorter in-hospital stay (Table 9.1). At the same time there was an increase in hospital medical staffing of 82%.

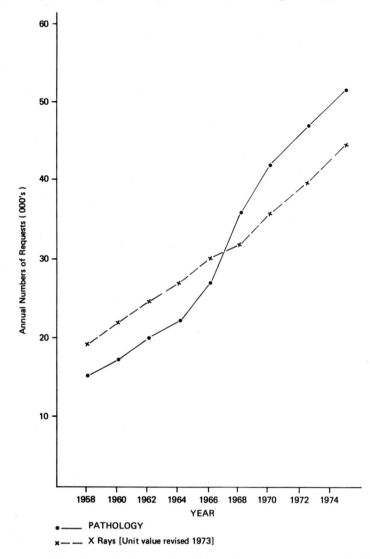

Figure 9.3 Use of pathological and radiological departments in British NHS hospitals (from DHSS, Annual Reports).

Table 9.1   Percentage changes in utilization of British NHS hospitals, 1949–74 (from DHSS, Annual Reports)

	Hospital beds in use	In-patients	In-patient stay	Out-patients (new)	Accident emergencies (new)	Medical staff
Per cent change	− 20	+ 70	− 50	+ 20	+ 100	+ 82

INTERNATIONAL DATA

There is a range in the patterns of utilization of hospitals in different countries. In my comparisons of health services in USSR, USA and UK (Fry, 1969) I found differences and similarities that are summarized in Table 9.2.

Table 9.2   Comparison of hospital resources and utilization data in USSR, USA and UK (from Fry, 1969)

	USSR	USA	UK
Hospital beds per 1000 population	9.6	8.9	9.6
Staff per 100 hospital beds			
Physicians	9	10	5
Nurses	38	59	56
Utilization			
Annual admissions per 100 population	20	15	10
Length of stay in hospital (days)	15	9	12

It seems that Russians are admitted to hospital more than are Americans or British and that they stay in longer. One reason may be that there are more general hospital beds. Of the 9.6 beds per 1000 only 0.93 were for psychiatric cases, the rest being classified as general. In the USA the proportions for the 8.9 beds per 1000 were 4.9 general and 4.0 psychiatric and in the UK for 9.6 beds per 1000, 5.6 were for general cases and 4.0 for psychiatric.

In the World Health Organization's study on health care (Kohn and White, 1976) the mean overall hospital admission rate (at least one overnight stay) was 11% for the twelve areas studied in North America, South America and Europe. In addition there were other patients treated as day cases and in North America this amounted to a further 4% who were hospitalized.

The range of overnight hospitalization, however, was from 15% in the six USA and Canadian areas, to 7% in Buenos Aires. Likewise, the mean overall length of stay in hospital was 12 days, with a low of 8 days in north-west Vermont, USA, and a high of 24 days in Lodz, Poland.

The rates of stay and hospitalization were related to availability of resources. Thus in areas where there were good facilities for short stay and day care in hospitals the length of stay was shorter than in areas where the traditions and facilities were geared more to long stay.

Where there were facilities for home nursing and home visiting by physicians the hospital admission rates were lower. They also were lower where individuals were responsible for paying all, or more usually part, of the hospital costs.

ROLES AND FUNCTIONS

The hospital is part of the fabric of health care. The hospital service cannot, and must not, be considered in isolation and separate from primary care services, from other community services and from self-care by the individual and the family. Each part has its own roles and functions to perform (see Chapters 1 and 2). To restate these:

Individuals and families must exercise their responsibilities for health maintenance, disease prevention, early diagnosis, self-care for minor and chronic disorders and co-operation and collaboration with professional services.

Primary care services must be available and accessible to the public. They must provide first-contact assessment, instant and long-term care in a continuing manner. They must be responsible for care of minor ailments, for most of the long-term care of chronic disorders and for the early diagnosis of major diseases. Their responsibilities must extend into prevention and health education in the community. They must co-ordinate the specialist community and hospital services for the good of their patients. They should protect the hospitals from conditions and patients who do not require hospital care.

Community services such as nursing, public health, social work and security have the important roles of providing care for the many social and similar problems that exist in every society. For optimal results and benefits the community services must work closely in collaboration with medical services.

Hospitals are specialist centres for specialists. They are buildings, clinics or groupings where special facilities and resources are placed to provide specialist care and services to populations for which they are responsible. The special resources include trained medical and para-medical staff as well as equipment.

Traditionally, hospitals provide facilities for persons to be nursed and cared for in their buildings because it is simpler and more economic to concentrate all the necessary resources in a hospital than to transport them to a private home. It should be remembered, however, that a century ago more major medical and surgical procedures were carried out in the patients' homes. When the late King George VI (of UK) had his pneumonectomy for lung cancer in 1952, it was carried out in an adapted room in Buckingham Palace and that is where Queen Elizabeth II was delivered of her four children (1948–60). Princess Anne had her first baby in 1977 in hospital.

Hospitals also provide facilities for specialist consultations (or are associated with clinics, or similar facilities, where such specialists work). In Britain they are termed out-patient services as distinct from in-patients who are admitted to the hospital.

Part of the equipment of a modern hospital are the investigative (or diagnostic) services, radiology and pathology. These are highly specialized and expensive and in an organized system should be available to all in the particular area served by the hospital; that is for primary care services as well as for hospital specialists. In the British NHS this is the pattern and the proportion of all requests for radiology by general practitioners is 10% of the total and for pathology 13%. The requirements for investigations in primary care are much less than in hospital practice.

The hospital also has responsibilities that should extend outside its own walls into the community. It should be concerned with the quality of primary medical and social care services in its area. The better they are and the more that can be cared for in the community outside the hospitals the better economic and medical use will be made of available resources. The hospital should support and collaborate closely with its local primary care and community services.

The local hospital is in a good position to act as the local educational centre for the local health profession and the public. Not only can health educational centres be set up at local hospitals but continuing education of physicians, nurses and other para-medical workers can be undertaken within the hospital.

TYPES OF HOSPITALS

Hospitals must serve the needs of the people and not vice versa. In a well-planned health care system different types of hospitals are needed at different population and geographical levels (see Figure 1.3, page 13).

The basic hospital must be a district hospital serving a population of between 100 000–250 000 persons, depending on the population density and transport access and facilities. Such a hospital will provide the first level of modern hospital care within the community. Its main work will be with the common hospital-type conditions in the community and it will require generalist orientated specialists.

In some communities with special traditions or geographical problems smaller community hospitals may be appropriate, staffed usually by local primary physicians. These tend to provide care for the less complex medical conditions in the community, such as chest conditions, disorders of ageing, terminal care and more minor surgical and gynaecological disorders. The population base for community hospitals is usually 10 000–50 000.

At a regional level with populations of 1–5 millions (depending on density) a regional hospital is necessary providing super-specialist units such as chest surgery, neurology and neuro-surgery, plastic surgery, radiotherapy, and others. These usually combine the roles of a local district hospital.

Although all hospitals must undertake teaching and training of their staff and local colleagues there must be teaching hospitals associated with medical schools that train and educate future physicians, nurses and others. It seems that in Europe and North America there is one medical school to about 2 million people.

These hospitals, or complexes of hospitals, must include demonstrations of work as community, district and regional hospitals, if they are to provide their students with a complete picture of health care.

Then there are special hospitals or units for certain disorders such as psychiatry, infectious diseases and long-term stay. These may be physically separate from district or regional hospitals or they may be a part of them.

PATTERNS OF HOSPITAL AND PRIMARY CARE ASSOCIATION

Since both hospital and primary care services are parts of a larger whole health care service there is need for them to work together. There are different ways of achieving this. There is no single best pattern. It has to be determined and achieved by many factors such as customs, traditions and expectations, incentives, resources and geography.

At least four patterns are recognizable.

1 There is the do-it-all situation which exists in a developing country or in an isolated community anywhere. That is, there is one (or more than one) physician, supported by para-medical auxiliaries, who is responsible for total care. He has a small community hospital and he provides primary and hospital care to that community. He refers more difficult cases to a district hospital, some distance away.

2 There is the situation that exists in North America and other places where primary physicians have hospital privileges and can provide care for their own patients when they are admitted to hospital. This includes care for medical, surgical and obstetric cases. There are usually recognized specialists on the staff of the hospital to whom the more difficult cases may be referred. Such hospitals are often small (less than 200 beds) and do not have resident junior hospital staff, the patients' medical care being shared between primary physicians and specialists.

The work is that expected in a district hospital with a predominance of surgery for piles, herniae, varicose veins, cysts and lumps, minor gynaecology, appendectomy, hysterectomy, tonsillectomy, cholecystectomy, mastectomy and perhaps for some other conditions, and peptic ulcers. Medical work will be for chest infections, asthma, heart failure, arthritis, myocardial infarction, strokes and patients being investigated and assessed. The hospital will be expected also to provide emergency room care.

There are advantages and disadvantages in such a system. The advantages are that the patients in hospital are cared for, at least partly, by their own physicians who know them; the primary physicians are in regular and continuing contact with the hospital and this serves as a form of continuing stimulous and education; and the specialists are in close communication with their colleagues in primary care. The disadvantages are that sometimes primary physicians may undertake care in which they are inexperienced because of their small hospital work-load; much time may be wasted in assisting at surgical operations carried out by surgeons; it may be uneconomic for specialists to work in such small units with small work-loads; and there is no good information on the quality of work in such a system.

3 In the UK, Europe and the Socialist countries where there is a clear division between primary care and hospital care. Once the patient is admitted to hospital he, or she, becomes the responsibility of specialists and their staff and the primary physician has no part in care during the hospital phase. Such a system requires good communications in both directions, to and from the hospital and primary care. Once the patient comes out of hospital he usually comes under the care of the primary physician.

There are disadvantages in the patient being removed from contact with his primary physician whilst in hospital, although often the latter is welcome as a visitor; the primary physician is cut off from intimate contact with the hospital; and there may be opportunities for off-loading cases from primary to hospital care. The advantages are care by specialists; in theory a better organized service; and also one of good quality.

4 There is a pattern which combines the last two and that is where the primary physician works in the hospital as a clinical (or medical) assistant. Here the primary physician will be employed as a member of a hospital specialist team or unit and provide care in the hospital for all, and any, patients and not only his own patients. This has the advantages in providing professional and educational contact between primary physician and hospital; it enlarges his special skills, experience and interests; it enables the primary physician not only to learn but also to teach the specialists and other members of the hospital staff; it provides the hospital with extra trained staff who are experienced and know the locality; and it provides patients with care by primary physicians within the hospital.

The disadvantages are that the primary physician is not providing care for his own patients; primary physicians are able to set aside only a few sessions each week to work in hospital; and their initial experience and training are uncertain.

In an ideal situation all primary physicians in an area should be offered such hospital assistantships on a rotating basis, that is a change of specialty attachment, say every 3 years, to allow others to serve.

FLOW AND ACCESS

A matter of considerable importance is the nature of flow and access to hospital by the public (Figure 1.4, page 14). There are two alternatives. In one, such as the British NHS, there is really a single portal of entry into the hospital service (apart from accident-emergencies, venereal disease and family planning clinics). Persons have to be referred by personal letter to a specialist in hospital. Such a referral system can work only if every person is entitled to a personal primary physician. Such a system also exists in Norway and Denmark and the Netherlands.

In the USA and Sweden there is an open access system where a person has direct and free access to specialists and to hospitals. Referral is not customary. In this system the hospitals have to be prepared and ready to provide primary and first contact care to any who seek it. There have to be large and busy emergency rooms and specialist clinics, both in hospital and elsewhere, are much busier than in the referral system.

In the USSR and in some large groups in the USA, the polyclinics combine the two and within the same group or clinic patients may select a primary physician or specialist as their first contact.

Finally, in a developing, or isolated, community there is a no-choice situation since there is only one physician or one unit to serve that area.

INFLUENCING FACTORS

The factors which will determine and influence the patterns of hospital care and organization are a mixture of social, administrative, medical and human.

Type of system

This is the major factor. It may be a total national health system such as in USSR or China where there is a single pattern. It may be a national health system with flexibility and independence as in the British NHS. It may be a national health insurance system as in Western Europe where the costs are covered but the relationships between patient, physician and hospital are relatively free. It may be a pluralistic system as in the USA where there is a mixture of all sorts. It may be a free-enterprise system where the individual is expected to meet the costs himself. All these will influence the patterns of hospital care.

Money and remuneration of physicians

This is a most important factor. If primary physicians receive higher remuneration for caring for patients in hospital and for carrying out hospital procedures, as in USA, then these physicians will be encouraged to admit their patients into hospital whenever possible. If primary physicians will lose fees by referring their patients to specialists such referrals will be low and patients will not be allowed free access to specialists.

Public and professional demands and expectations

In a democracy the form of health care will emerge from a compromise of public and professional wants and demands, but it will be slow in emerging and it will tend to be evolutionary and based on previous systems than completely new and revolutionary.

Local climatic and geographical facts

These may control completely what system can be realistic. Scattered and isolated communities with inclement climates cannot have similar services and systems to those of modern urban communities.

FACTS AND REALITIES

The nature of hospital and primary care

To restate the obvious:

There is one primary physician to 2500 persons.
There is one district hospital to 250 000 persons.
There are 100 primary physicians to one district hospital.

From these truisms certain facts flow.

Clinical content of primary and hospital care

In Table 9.3 an attempt is made to show numerically the clinical experience content of one primary physician and some specialists in the fields covered by the conditions noted.

Table 9.3 Number of selected conditions expected to be seen by a primary physician and a hospital specialist (from Fry, 1977)

Conditions	General practitioner per 2500	Hospital specialist per 250 000
Upper respiratory infections	600	? Nil
Acute chest infections	50	100
Asthma	30	50
Myocardial infarction	8	125
High blood pressure	5 (new)	75 (new)
	50 (continuing)	200 (continuing)
Cancer of lung	3	50
Cancer of breast	1	25
Cancer of large bowel	2	30
Strokes	5	120
Peptic ulcers	25	60
Acute appendicitis	5	100
Gall-bladder disease	3	30
Uterine fibroids	3	100
Backache	50	300
Diabetes	1 (new)	40 (new)
	10 (continuing)	250 (continuing)
Anxiety-depression	250	100

Staffing of a district health service

For a population of 250 000 Table 9.4 shows the approximate numbers of medical and nursing staff that may be expected (in the British NHS).

Table 9.4   Number of health staff in a district of 250 000 (from DHSS, 1977)

Community
General practitioners (primary care physicians)   100
Home nurses   60
Health visitors (public health nurses)   30
District midwives   10
Social workers   40
Medical secretaries-receptionists   200
Hospital
All specialists (consultants)   45
Junior hospital doctors   80
Nurses   150
Specialties
General medicine   6
General surgery   6
Psychiatry   5
Orthopaedics (and trauma)   3
Gynaecology   2
Paediatrics   2
Physical medicine and haematology   2
Ophthalmology   2
Ear, nose and throat   2
Pathology   5
Radiology   3
Others   7

These are numbers from the British NHS. Such an exercise to plot the staff is useful, even though there are great differences in other countries. Some of these differences are illustrated in Table 9.5.

Table 9.5   The number of surgeons in various countries for every one surgeon in the British NHS

	General	*Obstetrician-gynaecologist*	*Ear, nose and throat*	*Ophthalmic*
West Germany	3	2.5	4	4
USA	3	3	2	4
Australia	3	1.5	1	3
Norway	2.5	—	3	3
Canada	2	—	2	3
Belgium	2	1.5	3	5
Denmark	2	1	4	3
Italy	2	2	2	2
France	1	—	2	3
Sweden	—	—	3	2

The question may well be asked, what do these differences mean? Since the health of all these countries is not very different, do some have too many surgeons and others too few, or, are there some oddities in the nomenclature and the roles of these busy workers?

These differences in numbers of surgeons are reflected in their work. Thus appendectomy in West Germany is carried out three times as often as in the UK. Cholecystectomy is carried out six times as often in Canada as in the UK, and four times as often in the USA as in the UK (Bunker *et al.*, 1977).

Referrals by general practitioners to hospital

From published reports (RCGP, 1977) it seems that the referral rates of patients to hospital specialists has varied by ten-fold. Some practices report annual hospital referral rates of 2% of their population and others 26%.

The Second Morbidity Survey (OPCS, 1974) is the most extensive survey over 1 year and involved 119 physicians. Table 9.6 shows the rates of referrals for all the practices and the highest and lowest ranges bearing out the previous experience.

Table 9.6 Referrals to hospital by general practitioners (from OPCS, 1974)

Type of referral	Referrals per 100 of population		
	Mean	Highest	Lowest
In-patient	1.8 ⎱ 10.4	5.0 ⎱ 23.1	1.5 ⎱ 8.2
Out-patient	8.6 ⎰	16.1 ⎰	6.7 ⎰
Investigation	11.0	16.4	7.7

There is another important aspect. Do the referral habits alter in a general practitioner over the years? The answer is very much so. My own referrals to hospital specialists halved over 20 years (Fry, 1971) from a rate of 10.5% in 1951 to 5.0% in 1970 (Figure 9.4).

Clinical content of referrals

The groups of conditions that may be expected to be referred by one British general practitioner (with 2500 patients) are shown in Table

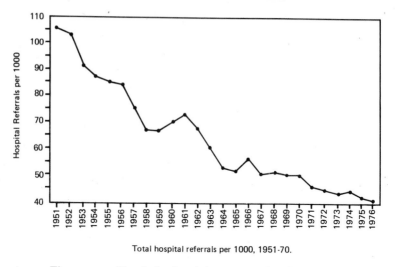

Total hospital referrals per 1000, 1951-70.

Figure 9.4   Hospital referrals in one practice (Fry, 1971).

9.7. These show that it is in the more general specialties that the general practitioner refers most of his patients.

Table 9.7   Numbers of patients referred in a year by a British general practitioner from a population of 2500 (from Loudon, 1977)

Clinical specialty	In-patients	Out-patients
Medical		
General medical	38	28
Paediatrics	12	10
Geriatrics	10	—
Chest	4	15
Dermatology	—	22
Cardiology	1	—
Surgical		
General surgical	52	52
Gynaecology	26	29
Orthopaedics-trauma	22	60
ENT	14	33
Urology	4	—
Neuro-surgery	1	—
Eye	5	30
Psychiatry	10	11
Maternity	44	39
Total	288	420

ISSUES AND IMPLICATIONS

The work of the hospitals and their relations with primary physicians and the community is of the greatest interest, importance· and significance to all who are concerned with health care. In this chapter I have looked at some aspects of hospital practice and there are some that require further probing and studies in depth. Some questions are appropriate.

1 What is a hospital for, in addition to its traditional roles of in-patient and out-patient care?

Should it not extend its interests, concern and involvement outside its own walls into the community and become concerned with prevention before the hospital episode and with after-care? The hospital episode is but a fleeting moment of time in the lifetime of any human being.

The hospital should become much more of a health centre than the present disease centre of a district community. At present it is too much of a hierarchical establishment, aloof and removed from the problems and needs of its local community. There are exceptions, but they are few.

The district hospital should provide the educational and research centre for its district. Such education should extend not only to the health professionals in the community but also to the public.

Research must include the problems of the community and its health outside, as well as inside, the hospital.

2 How much should the hospital be used?

The use and the costs of hospitals are increasing annually. How much more will they have to manage? How much of their work is really necessary? There is need for critical studies to be done to show what is useful and what is relatively useless in hospital work. The differences in operating rates on gall-bladders, tonsils, appendices, uteri and other organs are well known. How can a more rational approach to control of overuse be developed? Quality and quantity should go hand in hand in health care but quantity is often ahead of quality. Surely the principle of controlled trials must be applied more rigidly to procedures carried out in hospitals.

3 Staffing

The medical staff of British (and other) hospitals has doubled almost in the past generation. How much of this increase has really been necessary? This staff is still increasing through planned extension in the NHS by 4% each year. Is it really necessary? No one can tell unless and until the work of hospital doctors is analysed carefully.

4 The relationship between hospitals and primary care services

Where the referral system operates the work of the hospitals is in the hands of the primary physicians. There is an extraordinary range of difference in the referral rates of these physicians. Why and what can be done to reduce the rates of the high referrers? Surely what is required is more facts and data to show where and why the differences occur and then to use these to re-educate.

It probably is wrong to exclude the primary physician from the work of a hospital. There are different ways in which he may work in his local hospital. He should be encouraged to do so in ways which fit best to local patterns. These may differ in detail but the principle should be to encourage primary physicians to work in hospital with their specialist colleagues.

References

Ashley, J. S. A., Pasker, P. and Beresford, J. C. (1972). *Lancet*, **i**, 890

Bunker, J. P., Barnes, B. A. and Mosteller, F. (eds.) (1977). *Costs, Risks and Benefits of Surgery* (New York: Oxford University Press)

Department of Health and Social Security (DHSS). *Annual Reports* (1949–77) (London: HMSO)

Department of Health and Social Security (DHSS) (1977). *Personal and Social Services Statistics* (London: HMSO)

Fry, J. (1969). *Medicine in Three Societies* (Lancaster: MTP Press Limited)

Fry, J. (1971). *Lancet*, **ii**, 148

Fry, J. (1977). *Update*, **15**, 829

Fry, J. (ed.) (1977). *Trends in General Practice* (London: Royal College of General Practitioners)

Kohn, R. and White, K. L. (1976). *Health Care* (New York and London: Oxford University Press)

Loudon, I. S. L. (1977). In *Trends in General Practice* (London: Royal College of General Practitioners)

Office of Population Censuses and Surveys (OPCS) (1974). *Second National Morbidity Survey* (London: HMSO)

10
Community Social Services

The World Health Organization's definition of health is 'a state of physical, mental and social well-being and not merely an absence of disease'. The care provided by physicians and nurses deals predominantly with physical disorders and to a degree with mental problems but not very much with social pathology. The medical profession's contributions to health as defined by WHO must be a small proportion of the total expectations and needs of our society.

Health care must extend well beyond the clinical and medical confines of hospitals, clinics, health centres and practices. It has to move out into the community and involve the people themselves, health agencies of various forms and local and central governments.

The services expected by a modern society are more concerned with problems of living than with the more medical disorders. No longer are people so ready to accept the rigours and deficiencies of life. They expect help with provision of shelter, housing and clothing. They expect safe water, heating and food. They seek help with personal and family problems. They expect provisions to be made for care of their elderly, handicapped and mentally infirm. They expect help with medical care. They expect crime to be controlled, roads to be safe and transport to be available. They expect financial help when sick and when old.

In fact, the continuing trends are for individuals and families to expect to receive more from society then to give to it. It is difficult to draw lines and demarcations between the social and other components of health, and it is even more difficult to measure an individual's input into his community and also what he receives from it. Some individuals and families will inevitably receive more services than they are able to put in, but in all well-regulated and organized societies a balance between wants, services and needs has to be reached with the possible and available resources. Those whose needs are greater have to be supported by those who are fortunate enough not to require health and social care.

How these health, social and other community services are to be provided will depend on national systems of care. Yet all of us are facing dilemmas in striving to provide fair and equable care.

DILEMMAS IN COMMUNITY CARE

The dilemmas relate to questions that have to be asked and answered by each community and each nation. Whilst all caring societies must be ready and prepared to provide help for those of its members who are sick, handicapped, old and unable to work or care for themselves, they must also be ready to ask how much welfare is necessary and for whom. It is also appropriate to ask the question when does welfare become a disincentive? Whilst it is right that the needs of the needy must be met, it always will be difficult not to include some who prefer to accept social welfare assistance rather than to work and contribute to their society's needs. It is better to accept small numbers of such individuals than to make the real needy suffer.

How much should be provided and how many services should be made available? Who is to provide the services and how? Why are they being provided, with what results, and for whose good? When is enough enough? What community services are appropriate and useful and which are useless? To answer these questions there have to be built-in critical evaluations of what is being provided.

HISTORICAL

Kindness and concern are human characteristics that fortunately have been in evidence since time began. The extended family life of early history can still be seen in developing societies, where helping each other is a feature. Problems of village societies were, and still are, managed within the villages by responsible leaders and elders, often without recourse to outside assistance. More serious social problems – those of transposed and isolated families, of unemployment, of crime, of housing, of alcoholism and venereal disease – appeared with urbanization and industrialization and have been with us since. Since early times the Church and similar religious bodies have been concerned with welfare within the community. This stimulated voluntary and philanthropic works. In the nineteenth century hospital almoners became the first professional paid social workers, although even earlier there were unpaid amateurs.

The principles of social security and the state's responsibilities for individual and family welfare began to be set in the second half of the nineteenth century but it is only in the past 50 years and even more in the past 25 years that the concept of the Welfare State has emerged. Before World War I there were Friendly Clubs for working men to contribute to for providing assistance with medical costs and sickness. This was followed by the institution of health insurance in Prussia which spread to other parts of Europe and then to North America.

Now our Welfare Society provides cushioning against poverty, sickness, unemployment, personal and family crises and other special problems. To provide help social services have been developed and social workers have emerged as a fast-growing profession.

WORLD TRENDS

In the forefront in developing community services are Sweden, the Netherlands, France, West Germany, the USA, the UK, the USSR and the East European Socialist countries. Each has interpreted its own needs and patterns of welfare in keeping with their traditional national beliefs.

In the USSR and East Europe there is a clear and formalized system starting with local street or village health volunteers who are local people trained to provide advice, information and surveillance on public health and community social welfare. In China this has been similarly adapted to their local bare-foot doctors who in addition provide basic primary medical care. In West Europe and Scandinavia the systems are extensive and complex and often require guidance and experience in order to make the best use of them. The various parts of a social welfare system are often unconnected and widely separated both structurally and in their actions.

The needs for better organization and integration are present in all social security and welfare systems and an attempt to achieve this was made in the UK in the late 1960s and 1970s when separate departments of social services were set up in the areas of a reorganized National Health Service. The objectives were to provide better access to the public, to develop a more comprehensive and less rigid system of social care with emphasis on general casework by trained social workers who would be better able to mobilize available resources and to guide and direct their clients to the appropriate agency.

The results of the exercise have not been assessed in detail yet. There has been a great increase of social workers, their numbers have doubled in the past decade and a great deal more money has been spent and social services provided, but their cost benefits have not been quantified.

WHO DOES WHAT?

If the arrangements and organization of community services appear a confused muddle this is because they are in a state of confusion. By their nature and because of the problems that they are called upon to provide and the resources that are available to try and deal with them, these services lack some of the precision and definition of clinical medicine. Nevertheless some attempts must be made to show the extent and nature of the common social problems in a developed society and who is available to deal with them.

As noted already the basic needs of human beings are adequate and safe food, clean water, reasonable housing and clothing and enough money with which to purchase personal amenities. All people should be enabled to have such basic requirements plus access to medical and social care and support. Within every community there are certain vulnerable groups, families and individuals who will require special extra assistance. These include children, single-parent families, the aged, mentally sick and disabled and the physically handicapped.

Table 10.1 shows a more detailed presentation of the numbers of persons with social problems that may be expected to occur in a community of 2500 in the UK, the mean population base of a general practitioner.

A somewhat different classification is shown in Table 10.2 which shows the proportion of various problems that may be dealt with by a social worker in the UK.

Table 10.1 Social pathology in a population of 2500 in the UK (from Reedy, 1977)

Condition	Number of persons
Poverty (persons receiving supplementary social benefits)	150
Aged	
Over 65	360
Over 75	100
Children under 5	150
Single parent families (with children – 48)	27
Problem families (with children – 50)	10
Crime	
Found guilty of serious crime	17
Committed to prison	4
Unemployed	35
Bereaved	25
Divorce	5
Suicides	1 every 4 years
Drug overdoses	4
Alcoholics	20
Severe mental disorders	15
Severe physically handicapped	70

There is truly a vast army of persons who may be involved within the community in providing skilled and not-so-skilled care, support and advice for people in need. Table 10.3 shows who some of these

Table 10.2 Work of a social worker in the UK (from Hicks, 1976)

Conditions	Percentage distributions
Family and inter-personal problems	30
Psychiatric illness	20
Poverty, resource needs, housing and domestic assistance	20
Health and personal crises	15
Work and school problems	10
Others	5

may be and there must be many others. Altogether they may add up to about 1 person in 20 in the population caring or being prepared to provide care for those in social need.

Table 10.3   Groups in the UK who may be involved in community care

Medical profession
    Primary care team
    Hospital services
    Ambulance service
Pharmacist social work
    Social workers
    Home helps
    Meals-on-wheels service
    Residential staff of nursing and other homes
Police and courts
    Police
    Probation service
    Courts
Legal profession
    Lawyers
    Citizens' Advice Bureaux
Social security services
    Unemployment benefits
    Supplementary benefits (for poor)
    Retirement pensions
    Sickness benefits
    Attendance allowances (for those looking
       after handicapped or chronic sick)
Church
    Many persons and community services
Voluntary
    Self-help groups
    Philanthropic agencies
Elected representatives
    Local councillors
    Members of Parliament, etc.
Trade unions and professional organizations
The family, neighbours and friends

To provide a local appreciation of one part of the social and community services provided Table 10.4 shows the number of persons employed within the British NHS who provide care in a population of 10 000 which represents a typical group of general practitioners working together.

Table 10.4 Number of some community services and workers per 10 000 in the UK

Workers or service	Numbers
Primary care team	
General practitioner	4
Home nurses	2–3
Health visitors	1–2
Medical secretary-receptionists	8 (part-timers)
Social services	
Social workers	2–3
Home helps	16 (part-timers)
Meals-on-wheels	for 200 persons each week
Ambulance services	
Emergencies	2 per day
Other persons transported	10 per day

IMPLICATIONS

The implications of what has been discussed in relation to community social services are clear.

1 All human societies must accept that all their citizens must be able to have the basic needs for living. Most societies would agree that individuals and families are primarily responsible for providing these as rewards for their labours and input into their own societies, namely through pay and income.

2 There will be in all societies, groups and families of unfortunates and individuals who, for various reasons, need help and assistance from the more fortunate and some system of social security has to be provided. This may have started with help within an extended family or village but now with urbanization and industrialization the community and society has to accept this role.

3 There are agonizing dilemmas of who should be provided with what, why and how, and who should do the providing? There are immense complexities and difficulties when social welfare has to be provided and allocated. These difficulties must be accepted and dealt with as humanely as possible.

4 There is a need for constant questioning and experimenting to endeavour to prevent social problems whenever possible but at the same time to discover the best ways of helping those who need help.

References

Hicks, D. (1976). *Primary Health Care: A Review* (London: HMSO)

Reedy, B. L. E. C. (1977). In *Trends in General Practice*, J. Fry (ed.) (London: Royal College of General Practitioners)

Further reading

Goldberg, E. M. and Neill, J. E. (1972). *Social Work in General Practice* (London: Allen and Unwin)

11
The Primary Care Team

In the current anxiety over the structure, process and outcome of health care it has become evident to the planners who seek efficiency and to the economists who seek efficacy and value for money that primary care is an essential and an important part of health care. Even more important is the possibility that good primary care may serve not only to provide satisfactory and appreciated personal care for the individual and the family but also that it is a sound investment for limited funds and resources because it may protect the more expensive hospitals from inappropriate work (see Chapter 9).

The reawakening of interest in, and support of, primary care has been stimulated by the World Health Organization (Djukanovic, 1975; Newell, 1975) who sees in reorganized primary care the hopes for the most rapid improvements in health care.

Associated with support of primary care has been an examination of the roles and functions of those who provide the care. Spontaneously in many parts of the world the concept of a primary care team has been created and encouraged. No longer is the physician considered the most important member of the team. Related to the needs of primary care it may be that other workers may carry out equally important or even more important functions. The physician is the most expensive worker, his training takes the longest and his income is the highest. It makes sound sense to consider whether other less highly trained health workers may take over some of his traditional work.

Further reasons for the interest in the team are in the possible sharing of special skills and experience, in sharing of premises and resources and in better communication and liaison. The chief objectives must be to achieve better standards of health care at lower costs.

WORLD TRENDS

Traditionally the primary physician is still thought of as providing personal care on a one-to-one basis, often working on his own with little assistance or help from other health professionals. This is still the pattern in many parts of Western Europe, in North America, in South America, in Australia, in New Zealand and in South Africa. It is the stamp of primary care in a free-enterprise system where the physician is competing with others on a fees-for-services method of remuneration. However, even in the USA, Scandinavia, the Netherlands and more particularly in the UK, there have been moves towards team work in primary care. In the USSR sharing of primary care has been customary for many years. In the developing countries primary care is only possible at all on a team basis.

USA

Partly because of maldistribution of health services, geographically and socially, but largely because of the decline of organized primary care and the slow disappearance of the general practitioner and family physician, there has been interest in the past 10 years in creating primary care teams. Groups of medical specialists are not a valid and economic solution. The notable moves have been in the creation, or recreation, of nurse practitioners or medical assistants. These are specially trained para-medical workers who are expected to work in collaboration with and under the direction of physicians, to provide primary preventive, diagnostic and therapeutic care. The nurse practitioner is trained to work more independently as a first-contact worker in communities with few physicians, the medical assistants work with physicians in their offices or other centres.

Scandinavia

In outlying, remote and sparsely populated areas in Sweden, Norway and Finland nurses have, for many years, provided direct access primary care, working in close liaison and collaboration with district physicians who may be based some distance away.

Netherlands

The Netherlands is a densely populated urbanized country. Here primary care team-work has been developed between family physicians, midwives, social workers and nurses. Although each works as an independent professional, good working relations develop.

USSR

Only one-half of the USSR is urban, the other half is still rural. To provide care for all their 260 million team-work is essential (Fry, 1969).

In towns primary care is based on polyclinics and here primary physicians work closely with nurses both in the clinic and in the community. Liaison is also maintained with Saneped (public health) staff.

In the rural areas most primary care is provided by specially trained medical auxiliaries (feldshers) who are able to provide care for the common conditions (and to actively engage in disease prevention and health promotion) and to work closely with providing physicians who are based at a local community hospital. In addition to the trained professionals, physicians, feldshers and nurses, there is in every locality, village, farm, street or large living establishment a health volunteer. The health volunteer is a member of the public who receives some simple training in medical first-aid and public health and who has certain responsibilities in promoting good public health in his locality and in ensuring collaboration with the professionals.

UK

Impetus to the health team idea was given when it was decided to encourage the attachment of nurses, health visitors, midwives and social workers to general practice. These health workers are all employed by the National Health Service so that the general practices were not involved in any payment or financial loss. In addition, an arrangement was made that for any other secretarial or nursing staff employed by general practitioners, 70% of their salaries was to be reimbursed.

At present in over three-quarters of general practices there is a working association between general practitioners, nurses and health visitors. There is a long way to go before close team-work is achieved.

Developing countries

The most exciting examples of primary care team-work come from developing countries. The World Health Organization in two reports (Newell, 1975; Djukanovic and Mach, 1975) on achievements in China, Tanzania, Venezuela, Guatemala, India, Indonesia, Niger, Iran, Nigeria and Cuba, shows what can be done.

The emphasis is on self-help, on health by the people, on improvisation and adaptation of traditional and indigenous systems of care. The most important members, numerically, of the primary care team are not physicians, nurses, midwives or social workers but non-professional primary health care workers selected by the community from within the community. These workers should receive simple training in preventive measures; health and nutrition education; health and needs of mothers and children; use of simplified forms of medical and health technology; association with traditional forms of health care by traditional practitioners; and respect for the cultural patterns and needs felt by the consumers. These primary care health workers have to work in co-operation with doctors, nurses and midwives, whose training must be modified to enable them to work with and support the local communities.

FACTS IN THE UK

In the UK there are more general practitioners than there are nurses, health visitors, midwives or social workers (see Table 11.1). The work of attached nurses in the UK is relatively restricted: 47% is with basic nursing activities; 47% is with technical procedures; 6% is with social and health education. There is little evidence of any extension of the nurses' activities into doctors' roles.

The work of health visitors is concerned largely with helping mothers to bring up children under 5 (more than half of their time) and the rest is with elderly, mentally handicapped and some social problems. Once again the work is restricted and unimaginative.

The work of the social workers is in the same population as that cared for by general practitioners but collaboration between them is poor at present.

Table 11.1   Primary health team workers in England (from DHSS, 1977)

	Total number	*Group practice*
Population	46 million	10 000
General practitioners	20 400	4
Nurses	11 000 ⎱ 14 000	2 ⎱ 3
Nurses employed by GPs	3000 ⎰	1 ⎰
Health visitors	7500	1
Social workers	15 000	3
Home helps (part-timers)	88 000	15
Midwives	4855	1
Medical secretary-receptionists (part-timers)	50 000	8

AN EVALUATION

Allowing for the initial enthusiasm over the new concept of the primary care team it is necessary to make an evaluation of it in relation to the present state.

The advantages have been stated to be better care through providing services for previously unmet needs in areas where there have been no facilities or only poor facilities; better use of available professional manpower and technological resources through sharing and delegation between members of the team; better cost-effectiveness of the work carried out; better communications between the workers; and more satisfaction for the providers and the consumers. These are hypothetical beliefs that have not been tested and whilst they are desirable the mere setting up of teams and promotion of team-work will not achieve them unless there are strong decisions and directives aimed to achieve these objectives.

There are some disadvantages. The tradition of the solo independent private contractor primary physician is well established in many systems and care by a team may be difficult to accept by the consumers. Personal continuing care, one of the tenets of good primary care, will be made more difficult. Barriers of access for the patient occur when the physician is protected by secretary-receptionists, nurses and others placed as the new front-line workers. Problems of remuneration and payment both of the physician and his team arise in free enterprise and insurance systems. They are less likely in national health systems. Does the patient or agency pay the full fee for service if the care is given by a nurse or social worker, in lieu of the physician? There are legal problems in possible responsibilities for malpraxis charges. Is the physician responsible for his team? Leadership of the team is another problem. Should there be an overall leader in charge and if so must he be the physician? Nurses and social workers are increasingly unprepared to accept such conditions.

IMPLICATIONS

The concept of a primary care team is attractive hopefully to provide better health care with better value for money by making better use of available resources. It is relatively new in its full applications on wide local and national scales. Many good primary care units have included nursing, social and office staff and provided care through team-work with benefits to both consumers and providers. There is much less objective evidence to support such methods as national policies.

Before primary care team-work can be accepted as the pattern for the future there has to be evidence from well-planned pilot trials to show that better care is provided and that the exercise is more cost effective. There is the strong likelihood that such teams may lead to increased use of resources to provide care for medical and social problems and conditions that remain acceptable at present but which may create a vacuum of sophistication and a Pandora's box effect. For example, it may well be that the increased activities of the primary care team will lead to more demand from the aged and the handicapped, who seem to cope at present, for more home nursing and home help services, for more home baths, for more meals-on-wheels, for more telephones and for other social services and social security benefits. There have to be built-in safeguards and controls to guard against excessive demands and requests not only from the public but from the professional members of the team. There has to be sound evidence that team-work will lead to better health and not merely provide opportunities to spend more public money on dubious and unproven services.

A clear distinction has to be made between the conditions in developed and developing countries. The difference is partly one of quantity and quality. In developing countries with gross shortages of all resources the emphasis must be on providing any trained health care and quantity can be achieved most quickly by short courses of simplified health and medical care for selected volunteers from the community. In developed countries the accent must be on quality and better use of quality. The team must therefore set as its objectives, the best ways of making use of the skills and expertise of the various members of the team and being prepared to extend and expand the potential roles and functions of nurses and others.

FUTURE NEEDS

The concept of the primary care team is a reasonable one and it should be tried out on a planned trial basis everywhere. Within such trials there have to be clear objectives to measure and to evaluate any advantages and disadvantages.

Successful teams must accept close and harmonious collaboration among all members of the team who must regard each other as colleagues and professional equals. They must accept leadership, direction and control within the team and accept also the need for good communication between each other whilst maintaining professional confidentiality.

Above all new methods must be given opportunities of trial. The place of community health workers, who are drawn from the community and given a short training in simple health and medical matters, must be explored. In developing countries they are a most powerful factor in improving public health and public education. Developed countries may learn from the developing ones on the place of these new types of workers.

References

Department of Health and Social Security (DHSS) (1977). *Personal and Social Services Statistics* (London: HMSO)

Djukanovic, V. and Mach, E. P. (eds.) (1975). *Alternative Approaches to Meeting Basic Health Needs in Developing Countries* (Geneva: World Health Organization)

Fry, J. (1969). *Medicine in Three Societies* (Lancaster: MTP Press Limited)

Newell, K. W. (ed.) (1975). *Health by the People* (Geneva: World Health Organization)

Further reading

Reedy, B. L. E. C. (1977). *Trends in General Practice* (London: Royal College of General Practitioners)

12
Premises and Organization

In my travels, observing primary care services all over the world, I have seen good, and bad, care practised from huts in remote Africa, from collective farms in rural USSR, from adapted dwelling-houses in Western Europe and from superb purpose-built health centres and clinics in UK, USA, Canada, Sweden and Switzerland. This wide range of quality of premises raises questions of what premises, what organization and what resources are necessary for sound primary care?

To answer the questions, the nature of primary care has to be re-stated and its requirements examined.

THE NATURE OF PRIMARY CARE

In Chapters 2 and 3 a fuller analysis has been made and here a summary will suffice.

Primary care has to provide first-contact professional medical services in the community. To do this the unit has to be available and accessible to the community that it serves. Either it has to be within pram-pushing distance of walking patients, or there has to be reasonable public transport, or the community has to have available its own private transport or special transport must be provided.

The community served by a primary care physician in a developed country is relatively a small and static population of around 2500 persons for whom primary first contact and continuing care is provided. This means that the conditions and problems that are managed are minor (65% of all consultations), chronic (20%), and acute major (15%). In addition there are social, personal and family issues and problems to be dealt with.

Any organization of services, and any premises and resources that are provided should be related to these features.

Premises

The basic requirements are a consulting room for the physician, nurse or social worker; an examination room that may be combined with the consulting room or separate; an office for storage of records, for appointments and for other secretarial purposes; and a reception-waiting room (or area) for patients.

There may be refinements and additions depending on the roles that the primary care units undertake. Thus a treatment room and operating theatre may be necessary if the hospital is far away; diagnostic equipment may be needed for the same reasons; and there may be combinations of primary care and hospital services.

Types of organization

There is no single blueprint that is best. There are many variations on a common theme. The private practitioner may work alone from his own home or from adapted or purpose-built or group practice. The group may consist solely of primary care workers or it may include generalists, specialoids and specialists.

A health centre or medical centre may serve as the main community health unit with physicians sharing the premises with nurses, social workers and others to provide a wide range of services.

A polyclinic is the pattern in the USSR, and other socialist countries. These are purpose-built units that provide services for from 10 000 to 50 000 persons. These services include primary care by allocated specialoid paediatricians (for children) and therapists (for adults) and more specialist services by gynaecologists, surgeons, psychiatrists, ophthalmologists, dermatologists and others. There are diagnostic facilities, space for health education and for physical therapy and hydrotherapy.

In small and remote communities primary care units are often combined with a small community hospital and the same staff provide care in both.

Resources

The range of use of diagnostic investigations is wide and their usefulness has not been assessed, critically. My own annual rate of use of radiology is 7% of my practice population, or for 3% of all consultations. My annual rate for pathological investigations is 10% of the population or at 5% of consultations. These are low rates compared with the customs in North America where 1 in 3, or even 1 in 2, of all consultations may include referral for a laboratory test or X-ray.

From my own rate this means that for a practice of 2500, 175 persons will be X-rayed annually and 250 persons will have pathological tests. These are very small numbers to warrant special diagnostic facilities in a practice. Even with the much higher rates of North America the numbers per physician may be around 1000 a year. Even when, say, four or five physicians work together in a population of 10 000–12 000 the numbers will be insufficient for modern X-ray–pathology equipment. It requires a population of at least 100 000 to warrant such equipment.

It is uneconomic and wasteful to attempt to provide all these facilities in a small primary care unit. It is much better to provide them at a district hospital's diagnostic units and arrange to transport the specimens and/or the patients. The more simple tests on blood and urine can be carried out at the primary unit and so can simple straight X-rays of limbs and the chest, if distances from the local district hospital make it difficult of access. Alternatively, there is no reason why centralized diagnostic facilities should not be provided outside a hospital, by private or public agencies, for populations of adequate size.

The range of therapeutic facilities in primary care units will depend on how much the physicians are prepared to do and also on the extent of collaboration with hospitals and other units. Unless the local hospital is close by and provides facilities for minor surgery and trauma, then primary care units must have resources to carry out minor surgical and medical procedures and to provide care for minor trauma. For this to be done simple radiological, ECG and pathology facilities should be available.

Local geography and population density will influence the need for hospital beds as part of the primary care facility. In cities there is no need to have bed facilities available but in outlying, remote and sparsely populated areas there is a good case for a small number of hospital-type beds to be available as part of the primary care resources, in which the physician and his team can care for those patients who do not require transport to a district hospital.

ORGANIZATION

Efficient satisfactory organization in primary care will depend on meeting the needs and expectations of consumers and providers.

The consumer wants ready access and availability and short waits for personal care by a physician whom he knows. For this to be achieved the primary care unit has to be within a reasonable distance for the transport facilities available. It may have to be within walking distance or within the scope of public or private transport facilities.

Telephone links must be available and efficiently and courteously operated. The telephone is used in some parts of the world as a most important source of communication and consultation in primary care.

A well-run appointment system will have advantages to patients and doctors. There should be short waits for the patient to see the doctor and the doctor should be able to plan his work. There are problems that must be anticipated and avoided. An appointment system must not be allowed to become a barrier between patient and doctor. In primary care the longest waiting time for an appointment must never be longer than one day. The essence of good primary care is ready availability of a doctor or the team, and the patient expects advice and help when he, or she, feels the need.

It is not possible for a doctor to be available continually on a 24-hour basis. There have to be provisions for some alternative out-of-hours cover on a rota or a deputizing system. Ideally the cover should be a rota system shared between a small number of primary physicians in that area. Other systems include deputizing services by doctors who work in hospitals or elsewhere and emergency care provided by accident-emergency departments of hospitals.

Home visiting should be a part of primary care. Some patients have to be treated in their homes by the primary care team for short- or long-term illnesses and help and facilities need to be provided for this to be possible. Home visiting also enables information to be obtained on the family and individual home conditions.

Certain groups and certain disorders are best cared for through specially organized clinics. Thus child care and antenatal care are usually provided in this way but there is also a good case for providing special sessions for general screening, for family planning, for diabetes, for high blood pressure, for the elderly and for others. These special clinics are justified only if there are sufficient numbers of persons within these groups to justify the arrangements. Thus it is not reasonable to organize a clinic for 3–4 diabetics, but it is so for 5–10 expectant mothers.

As special services, arrangements may be made for health education and other preventive exercises to be carried out by the primary care team.

RECORDS

Medical records are an essential and important part of all forms of medical practice. They serve to record clinical and social data, to note progress and to act as sources for evaluation of the working of the health care system. Medical records have to be designed and created to meet these needs. They have to be legible, they have to be meaningful and they have to be appropriate for their purpose.

Of recent years there have been many attempts to change the format and content of medical records for various reasons. New data-processing technology has created an interest in the use of such technology for primary care. Dissatisfaction with international medical nomenclature has led to attempts to create new approaches based on problem orientation rather than on specific diagnostic labels of diseases. Almost every month there are reports of new systems of record-keeping for primary care. This is confusing and leads to uncertainty and apprehension. What is required is simplicity and clarity in medical recording and the development of records that will serve limited purposes and not attempt too much.

Whilst there have to be some international and national agreement on the basic contents of medical records, it is right that individual physicians and others be allowed individual flexibility to arrange and keep these records as they wish. Any good system of primary care records should serve as an instant guide to the individual's personal background, to his medical and social history to-date and to any special notable previous events, sensitivities or other alerting facts.

The basic data set should include: personal data; summary sheet (a card); on-going notes; any special individual features. Data that is required to provide answers to special operational or clinical questions has to be obtained through special records and special collection. It is not possible to create and keep a single all-purpose medical record that can be used by all to answer all possible questions. Each system has to evolve its own basic records but each individual physician and team has to be allowed freedom to keep his or her records in his or her own way.

TRENDS IN THE UK

Data from the UK shows the trends of organization over the past 25 years. Figure 12.1 shows the trend that the number of general practitioners is increasing in relation to the population.

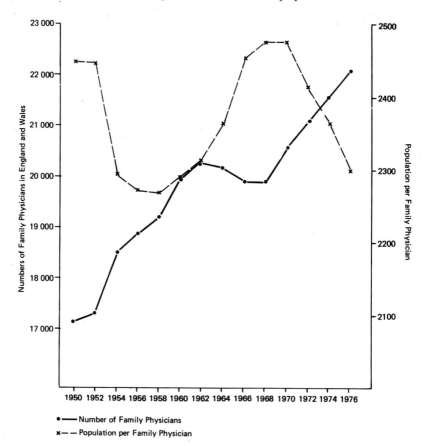

Figure 12.1 Numbers of general practitioners and their ratio per population in the UK (from DHSS, Annual Reports).

The proportion of women general practitioners in the UK is increasing, is now 13% and is likely to reach 25–30% over the next decade.

In the British NHS almost 20% of general practitioners are now foreign medical graduates, chiefly from Asia. Their proportion is likely to increase to 30% before falling.

There has been a great change in the organization of general practice in the NHS (Table 12.1). Whilst in 1951 almost one-half (43%) of general practitioners were in solo practice and only 1% worked in groups of five or more, now less than one in five (17%) are solo and 19% work in practices of five or more partners.

The numbers of general practice units in 1951 in England and Wales was 15000. In 1976 there were 8620 units. The trend has been for more general practitioners to work together in shared premises.

Another trend has been in the building and opening of purpose-built health centres, that is units that provide premises not only for doctors but for nurses, health visitors, social workers and others.

Before 1948 there were only four health centres in Britain. Now there are over 1000 with some 70–100 new health centres opening each year over the past 5 years. Of the British population 20% now receives primary care from health centres. On average, each health centre houses five general practitioners and associated primary health workers providing care for 12000 to 15000 people. There are much larger health centres serving as a base for over 30 doctors but these are exceptions in special densely populated areas. The pattern is for the smaller type of health centre closely linked to the local district hospital which provides diagnostic facilities and specialist services.

Table 12.1 Percentages of general practitioners in partnerships in the NHS in England and Wales (from DHSS, Annual Reports)

Year	Size of practice (number of physicians)						Total number of general practitioners
	Solo	2	3	4	5	6+	
1951	43	38	13	5	1	0	17 202
1961	31	34	21	9	3	2	20 005
1971	20	23	27	17	8	5	20 600
1976	17	21	25	18	10	9	21 667

As noted in Chapter 11, most (80%) of general practices in the UK have attached nurses and health visitors who work in collaboration with the doctors.

IMPLICATIONS

The chief implication is that premises and organization must be related to the nature and to the true requirements of primary care. There is no need for elaborate, sophisticated or expensive premises and equipment. The true needs are modest. More expensive diagnostic and therapeutic facilities are best shared with local hospitals or other private agencies.

Reference

Department of Health and Social Security (DHSS). *Annual Reports* (London: HMSO)

Further reading

Fry, J. (ed.) (1977). *Trends in General Practice* (London: Royal College of General Practitioners)

13
Prevention and Postponement

The ultimate goal of good health care must be a long, happy, active, useful and trouble-free (from physical, mental and social problems) life for as long as possible. This goal has to be shared among public, professional and individual responsibilities. Each has an important role to play and none can succeed working and striving alone.

Since death is an inevitable end to life the goal of good health care must be qualified and aim to postpone death for as long as possible by preventing unnecessary disease and suffering.

ACHIEVEMENTS

We are living longer than ever before. The biblical 'three score and ten years' of alloted life is now being achieved more than ever before. Life expectancy at birth in developed countries is now around 70 years for a baby boy and over 75 years for a baby girl.

We have achieved quantity of life but not quality. People do not appear to be more happy or to suffer less from disorders of stress and unhappiness. There is much social and mental distress everywhere. Nowhere has health in the World Health Organization definition been achieved.

A closer look at life expectancy tables shows that the great improvements have been achieved largely because of safer childbirth and safer childhood. The life expectancy of adult men over 45 has not increased much and may actually have fallen in some countries. This is due to the effects of unhealthy living, self-abuse and environmental stress and hazards and it is here that exist the challenges to prevention of disease and postponement of death, or prolongation of life.

It is useful yet again to remember that the major achievements in better health have been the result of progress in public health and social conditions rather than medical miracles and advances. Safer water, cleaner, more wholesome and more plentiful food, better housing and clothing, and safer work and safer roads created improved health long before the introduction of immunization, antibiotics, replacement surgery, psychotropic drugs and advances in molecular biology.

There will need to be much more effort from the medical profession in general and from individuals in particular in the future to improve health and to prolong life.

WHAT IS PREVENTABLE AND HOW?

The major killers today in modern developed societies are heart diseases, cancer, strokes, respiratory diseases, accidents and various other manifestations of self-abuse such as suicide and alcoholism. The major causes of morbidity in our societies are respiratory infections, emotional disorders, skin rashes, various psychosomatic disorders of function, including sexual problems and a variety of other disturbances in satisfactory life performance. The great problem is which of these diseases and disorders are preventable and how?

It is necessary to know much more about their nature and causes and even more about the usefulness or uselessness of the various attempts at prevention. As of now there are more general than specific possibilities for improvements. In the public field there have to be continuing efforts to improve the quality of life through even better social conditions in the home, at work and on the roads. The environment has to be made safer.

The medical profession has to continue to research into possible ways of controlling disease and improving life but these have to be tempered by the need to be certain that the techniques employed are effective and safe. Early diagnosis and applications of selected and proven therapies are well-tried methods but there is no good evidence that wholesale and mass screening of populations or blind regular and routine medical check-ups of individuals are useful exercises. The medical profession has also special opportunities to practise health education both in the public and in the personal fields.

It must be accepted, however, that the chief hopes for preventing disease, improving health and prolonging life are in the hands of individuals themselves. The rules of health are well known and scarcely need constant repetition. Yet their application seems to be difficult, if not impossible, for many people. These rules simply are to:

1 eat less and keep weight at an optimal level;
2 control alcohol consumption to a safe level;
3 avoid prescribed and non-prescribed drugs unless really necessary;
4 take regular physical exercise;
5 do not smoke;
6 take care to avoid accidents;
7 ensure enough sleep;
8 avoid unnecessary stresses.

There is nothing dramatic or new about these but their personal application would do much to improve health and to prolong life.

IMPLICATIONS FOR THE FUTURE

In theory the physician and his para-medical colleagues should devote much time in preventive work endeavouring to prevent diseases, accidents and problems from ever occurring. Much of this work already goes on with immunizations, in normal personal clinical work with early diagnosis and advice on care, life styles and on avoidance of harmful habits, and in professional and public committees and activities arrived at community actions.

There are dangers, however, in overaction by the physician and his team that may lead to over-reaction by the individual and the public. The individual is liable to resent constant attempts to make him alter his or her life-style, even if it may lead to better health. Take the case of smoking. Every person knows the dangers of cigarette-smoking, yet the numbers smoking and the number of cigarettes smoked have scarcely changed. Repeated efforts and attempts by a physician to make a patient give up smoking may lead to a loss of that patient. He will seek a physician less aggressive in his health education approach. Prevention is good in theory but difficult in practice.

14
Education and Learning

Education is a continuum that starts at birth and finishes, incomplete, at death. Life and living are general educating processes. Medical education is a specific process of education that is added to the student's life experience. It too has to be a continuum. Whilst it may be useful to subdivide medical education into undergraduate, graduate, vocational and continuing postgraduate phases, they should not be considered independently. Each contributes to the learning process, albeit with different goals and different educational techniques.

The case has been made for primary care to be recognized as a special field requiring special education and training because of its special core of knowledge and special skills. It is now proposed to examine some of the implications of this and to examine some of the trends.

CHANGING TRENDS IN MEDICAL EDUCATION

Medical education has become an increasing special field of its own. Medical educationalists are appearing and are laying down ground rules and are encouraging more and more complex methods of learning and teaching. Learning and teaching machines are being developed.

Audio-visual aids, well beyond the blackboard and chalk, are part of the paraphernalia of all schools, colleges and universities. Electives and groups are in fashion. Traditional exams are being replaced by less threatening (to the teacher as well as to the student) methods of continuous assessment. These tests that are being taken by students are based on answers to hundreds of multiple-choice questions. Traditional essays requiring more thoughtful presentations are considered ineffective as tests and students may graduate from medical schools without ever being required or encouraged to present any papers, reports or essays in a form or language that test their abilities in this form of communication.

Student power, the student's voice and the student's participation in curriculum planning, in administration and in selection of new students have been incorporated into schools, colleges and universities. It is said that there have been benefits and advantages from this process of consumer involvement in education but the advantages lack any strong objective support.

In spite of all these changes and activities in medical education there is no evidence that the final product of the doctor, be he in general family practice or in specialist consultant practice, is very different from his father, or even his grandfather. What is evident is that the changes have increased greatly the cost of medical education, led to much more complexity and created unease and uncertainty among many teachers.

THE PURPOSE OF MEDICAL EDUCATION

The purpose of medical education, surely, is to produce a doctor who is so trained and educated that he can fit into the system of health care in which he works and to provide sound care and service to his patients and at the same time meet his responsibilities to his community, his profession and the health care system. It has to be recognized that the trained doctor must accept some restriction of complete clinical freedom to meet the needs of the system in which he works. His medical education therefore must have as its objectives not only the production of a basic doctor but also one trained to take his place in his, or her, society and in that society's system of health care.

It has generally been believed that the purpose of undergraduate medical education is to train a young man, or woman, in the basic sciences, in scientific medicine and in behavioural sciences to be able and ready to apply these in modern scientific health care. Science is the operative emphasis. There is continuing competition from all the many sciences that exist in a modern medical school for a slot in the curriculum. The modern medical student becomes befuddled and confused by the science that he is taught, which scarcely fits him for the pseudo-scientific world outside when he leaves his medical school.

It may be that there have to be a small number of alternative tracks in the medical schools of the future that relate more closely to the needs of society and local communities than to the worship of gods of medical science and technology. Why should there not be a route for future primary care physicians where there will be more emphasis on applications of science, technology, behaviour and epidemiology to clinical practice for those interested in such work and another for those keen on the less applied scientific and techno-logical disciplines? – always allowing opportunities to switch routes.

BASIC UNDERGRADUATE MEDICAL EDUCATION

Whatever its format and contents the purpose of undergraduate medical education must be to produce a doctor who is ready and prepared to undertake the next stage of his education, that of graduate vocational training in his chosen specialty. Whatever his (or her) future career, it is important that he (or she) receives some teaching on primary care during the undergraduate period. It may be more important for those physicians who do not enter primary care to receive such education than for those who do, so that they may understand something about the place, the nature, the roles and the problems of primary care in the setting of the health care system.

Since more than one-half of all medical students will eventually serve as primary care physicians (Figure 14.1) this is another reason why possible tracks for primary care should be considered in some medical schools at least.

Each medical school must have a department of primary health care. Such departments should be associated with general district hospitals. They must teach both within the hospitals as well as in the community. They must teach on patients who are in hospital beds and who attend the out-patient departments to show why they are there, what are the problems and what services and care will be needed when the patient leaves hospital. As well as teaching on what happens in primary care there is necessity to concentrate on the interface between primary care and hospital care. There is need to emphasize the difference between the transient and instant snap-shot picture type of clinical situation in the hospital and the continuing movie picture of disease and its care in primary care.

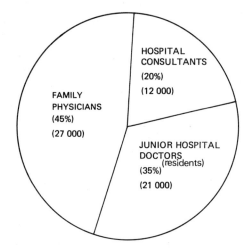

Figure 14.1 Proportion of medical students becoming primary care physicians in the British NHS.

Teaching by the Department of Primary Care must take place at all stages of the undergraduate curriculum and it should take place in shared time collaboration with other departments in the hospital with specialist clinicians, in the medical school with the non-clinical subjects, and in the community with medical and social practitioners.

The department of primary care must fulfil its research obligations as well as those of service and teaching. There is tremendous need for clinical and clinical epidemiological and clinical operational studies. Primary care is a new specialty that is lacking a sound core of knowledge based on research and experiment.

VOCATIONAL TRAINING

Primary care, general practice or family medicine have to have a period of special training in residency (USA) or vocational training (UK) programmes. Such programmes exist and are growing.

They are generally 3 years long, 2 years in special hospital appointments and 1 year in primary care. The training experience is supple-
mented by tutorials, day-release courses, projects, assessments and
examinations.

In the UK one-half of all future entrants into general practice are
now undertaking non-compulsory vocational training. From the
1980s it will become mandatory for all general practitioner principals
to undertake an approved 3-year vocational training programme.

CONTINUING EDUCATION

Once in an established specialty the doctor must continue with his
own personal continuing education for as long as he remains in
practice. It is best that he acquires the habit early and that he
maintains it with an obsessional regularity.

There are many ways of continuing learning and education and
in keeping up to date. The most traditional, the most widely used
and possibly the most useful is by reading – by reading professional
journals, books and reports. For the primary physician the most
useful reading material are review articles and reports from his own
specialty. Learning by doing is what we all do but this is made much
more useful if such doing can be recorded and analysed in some
simple form in order to provide opportunities to examine and study
the results in a constructive manner and especially if it can be
compared with the experiences of other colleagues.

Lectures, courses, group-discussions, audio-visual aids and other
methods appeal to some but whatever extra is done there has to be
a regular daily and weekly base of reading, discussion and analysis.

IMPLICATIONS

It is possible to make 'too much of a meal' of medical education. It
has become a sophisticated academic department in some medical
schools. It is an old process with many new ideas, methods and
machines. The new have to be tried out but the old well-worn and
accepted methods must not be rejected and thrown out.

There are no alternatives to the old hard slog of self-instruction
through reading, learning and 'inwardly digesting' what we have
to know. We can be helped in all of these. The reading material may

be made more appropriate, more attractive and more digestible. The learning process may be made easier by good teachers. The inward digestion however remains a highly personal exercise.

Further reading

Nuffield Provincial Hospitals Trust (1968). *Screening in Medical Care* (London: Oxford University Press)

15
How Much Care?
Present State and
Future Needs

Although we live selfishly and myopically in our own countries, we are members of one world, one human race, that has more similarities than differences. This applies also to health and health care. The attainment of health and its maintenance are common human goals and the provision of the means through health care is now an acknowledged human right.

Although there is no single best-buy system of health care that can be applied to every country, all systems of health care are part of the social structure of a country and must be part also of the culture, history, economics, geography and politics of that country. Nevertheless, within every system of health care there are, as has been demonstrated in Chapter 1, certain inevitable common levels of care and administration that have common roles and tasks to carry out.

All systems of health care, whatever their finer differing points of detail, now face the same common problems and dilemmas of attempting to match wants, needs and resources.

COMMON PROBLEMS AND DILEMMAS

Because of the insoluble equation of health care, where expectant wants always will be greater than assessed needs which will always be greater than available resources, and, because of the constant vacuum of sophistication, where wants never will be fully satisfied there is a huge bottomless pit into which more and more health care resources are being pitched.

The common dilemmas are how to control the three parts of the equation. How can wants be discouraged? How can needs be fairly and justly assessed? How can resources be best utilized? These are questions that have to be asked and answered in all health care systems. There are no ready and easy answers. We have to engage in detailed studies and we have to learn from one another.

Allied to these dilemmas are others. Since an insoluble equation of health care will be inevitable in the foreseeable future everywhere there have to be priorities in the use of resources and there has to be rationing. There have to be controls and directives. There have to be gate-keepers controlling entry into care.

The key questions that follow are, how should the priorities be allocated and to whom, and what forms of control should be used? In free-enterprise systems resources are utilized not according to needs but rather on the basis of who can best afford to pay the medical bills. If this is considered to be inequitable and inappropriate then alternative schemes must be developed.

COMMON AIMS

The common aims in our present economic world situation must be to make the best use of resources that always will be limited and which always will have to be shared out between many wants and needs. The challenge facing all health care systems must be to make decisions on how much care is necessary. There are three subdivisions to this question:

1 What care is effective? That is, what care is worth giving, what is useful and what is useless?

2 What care is efficient? That is, what are the best methods and techniques of carrying out the care?

3 What is good-quality care? That is, having set objective standards of excellence, that are in keeping with available resources, how does the care given match up to these standards?

THE PRESENT STATE

From these general attitudes let us turn to the present state of health care all over the world. We have been, and still are, in a booming expensive market of health care. Our targets have been set high. Health has been the goal, the aim, the objective, the target, the mirage for everyone. Health that is, as defined by the World Health Organization – a state of complete physical, mental and social well-being and not merely an absence of disease. Such an objective is unrealistic and unattainable by most persons for any length of time. It is a false hope for many and creates an explosion of unmet wants that cannot possibly be met in any system. Unmet wants lead to frustration and dissatisfaction. It is wrong to hide the truth from the public. Whilst it may be politically expedient sometimes to make rash promises, it never is right to do so in planning a health care system.

Another false illusion is to suppose that money alone can buy health. This is quite wrong both in the individual and in a public system. Personal wealth cannot, and never will, buy good health. It may make scant resources available but it will not prevent, or cure, disease alone. The same applies to new-rich nations. Buying and installing the latest and most expensive medical technologies with oil revenues cannot buy health for the people unless much more is done as well to improve the quality of their lives and living.

Much of the care and treatment given to sick people now is just as senseless and useless when it is given by formally trained physicians as it is by traditional healers or plain quacks. The facts are that in spite of the emphasis on science and scientific methods in medical schools and academic bodies, scientific principles seem to evaporate and are strikingly missing from the care being given to the masses of sick people in all parts of the world today. Much of modern medical care lacks sense and sensibility.

The further one moves away from the temples of medical science the more difficult it is to apply scientific principles and the more difficult it is to find much justification in some of the treatments given. This criticism is not only for the physician, but it relates very much to the pandered over-expectations created in a public demanding of care for conditions for which no care is useful.

Costs of medical care are escalating everywhere. They cannot go on at the present rate. There will have to be controls of the factors that make up the costs – physicians' fees, hospital bills and the rest.

There is the clarion-call being sounded of prevention rather than cure. This is fine and much can be done in developing countries to improve the quality of life that is dependent on good food, clean water and adequate housing and clothing, but in developed countries prevention, whilst still full of hope, is associated with personal and group behaviour habits, and prevention of diseases of developed societies require such mundane, but apparently excessively difficult, actions, such as stopping smoking, reducing alcohol, avoiding stress, eating less and exercising more. Whose are the responsibilities for better health in such circumstances?

FUTURE NEEDS

What of the future? The challenges are becoming clear – to make the best use of available resources for appropriate needs and to control unnecessary and unproven wants.

High priorities are two characteristics that are rare in modern life – honesty and humility.

Honesty is the challenge to state clearly and forcefully that there are strict limitations to the scope of modern medicine. We still can only 'cure sometimes, relieve often and comfort always'. The medical profession is prone to the ALG syndrome (Acting Like God) and it is most hard and difficult to admit sometimes to one's own and one's profession's limitations, even in these days of high technological achievements.

Humility must follow. All who are offered the opportunities to provide care and comfort for our fellow men must strive constantly to remain humble, as well as honest. There is so much unknown in medicine. Unknown causes, unpredictable course, and uncertain management.

Awareness that new is not always best and that old is not always bad is underlined by Sir Robert Hutchinson's prayer:

From ability to leave well alone,
From too much zeal for what is new and contempt for what is old,
From putting knowledge before wisdom,
Service before art, cleverness before common sense,
From treating patients as cases,
And, from making the care of a disease
More grievous than its endurance,
Good Lord deliver us.

148

Facts and data

In spite of the emphasis on science in medical schools there is a great lack of scientifically reliable facts and data on the efficacy of the treatment of common diseases and common problems and on the ways in which resources are used. There must be constant data available based on randomized controlled trials to give guidance on what is therapeutically useful and what is useless. We must know how available services are being used and misused if corrective steps can be taken. Reliable facts and data must be used to inform and educate the general public and the medical profession to use health services better.

Actions

All health care systems must be planned and organized nationally. The costs and complexities of modern medical care are so great now that they are well beyond the reach of normal private purses. There have to be government or quasi-government involvement and assistance in providing the resources and the money.

A sound health care system must have carefully planned policies based on reliable intelligence, facts and data. It must be able to exercise controls and directives and take steps to try and maintain high standards. This is not easy faced with a medical profession that treasures clinical professional freedom, a public seeking more and more care and costs that are ever rising.

These common difficulties create challenges for leadership – professional leadership and public leadership.

Further reading

Fry, J. (1969). *Medicine in Three Societies* (Lancaster: MTP Press Limited)

Kaser, M. (1976). *Health Care in the Soviet Union and Eastern Europe* (London: Croom Helm)

King, M. (1966). *Medical Care in Developing Countries* (London: Oxford University Press)

McKeown, T. (1976). *The Role of Medicine* (London: Nuffield Provincial Hospitals Trust)

Mahler, H. (1975). *Lancet*, **ii**, 829

Morley, D. (1973). *Paediatric Priorities in the Developing World* (London: Butterworths)

Wadsworth, M. E. J., Butterfield, W. J. H. and Blaney, R. (1971). *Health and Sickness: the Choice of Treatment* (London: Tavistock)

Index